# CARDIAC TOXICITY
# AFTER TREATMENT FOR
# CHILDHOOD CANCER

# CARDIAC TOXICITY AFTER TREATMENT FOR CHILDHOOD CANCER

**Editors**

**J. Timothy Bricker,** M.D.
Department of Cardiology
Texas Children's Hospital
Houston, Texas

**Daniel M. Green,** M.D.
Department of Pediatrics
Roswell Park Cancer Institute
Buffalo, New York

**Giulio J. D'Angio,** M.D.
Department of Radiation Oncology
Hospital of the University of Pennsylvania
Philadelphia, Pennsylvania

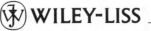

**WILEY-LISS**

A JOHN WILEY & SONS, INC., PUBLICATION
New York • Chichester • Brisbane • Toronto • Singapore

**Library of Congress Cataloging-in-Publication Data**

Cardiac toxicity after treatment for childhood cancer / editors, J.
    Timothy Bricker, Daniel M. Green, Giulio J. D'Angio.
      p.  cm.
    Includes bibliographical references and index.
    ISBN 0-471-59107-6
    1. Tumors in children—Chemotherapy—Complications—Congresses.
  2. Tumors in children—Radiotherapy—Complications—Congresses.
  3. Cardiovascular toxicology—Congresses. 4. Anthracyclines-
-Toxicology—Congresses. I. Bricker, J. Timothy. II. Green,
Daniel M. III. D'Angio, Giulio J. (Giulio John), 1922-  .
    [DNLM: 1. Antibiotic, Anthracycline—adverse effects—congresses.
2. Heart—drug effects—congresses. 3. Heart—radiation effects-
-congresses. 4. Neoplasms—in infancy & childhood—congresses.
5. Neoplasms—therapy—congresses. 6. Radiotherapy—adverse
effects—congresses. QZ 266 C267 1993]
618.92'12071—dc20
DNLM/DLC
for Library of Congress                  93-10065
                                       CIP

**The text of this book is printed on acid-free paper.**

# Contents

# Contributors

**Frank M. Balis,** M.D.
Pediatric Branch, National Cancer Institute, National Institutes of Health, Bethesda, MD 20892 [115]

**Gerald Barber,** M.D.
New York University, New York, NY [87,95]

**Robert S. Benjamin,** M.D.
M.D. Anderson Cancer Center, Houston, TX 77030 [109]

**Stacey L. Berg,** M.D.
Pediatric Branch, National Cancer Institute, National Institutes of Health, Bethesda, MD 20892 [115]

**Margaret E. Billingham,** M.B., B.S., F.R.C.Path.
Department of Pathology, Stanford University School of Medicine, Stanford, CA 94305 [17]

**J. Timothy Bricker,** M.D.
Department of Cardiology, Texas Children's Hospital, Houston, TX 77030 [ix,1]

**Edward B. Clark,** M.D.
Department of Pediatrics, The Cancer Center, University of Rochester Medical Center, Rochester, NY 14642 [103]

**Steven D. Colan,** M.D.
Department of Pediatrics, Harvard Medical School, Boston, MA 02115 [45]

**Giulio J. D'Angio,** M.D.
Department of Radiation Oncology, Hospital of the University of Pennsylvania, Philadelphia, PA 19104-4283 [ix]

**Sarah S. Donaldson,** M.D.
Department of Radiation Oncology, Stanford University Medical Center, Stanford, CA 94305 [35]

**Michael S. Ewer,** M.D., M.P.H.
M.D. Anderson Cancer Center, Houston, TX 77030 [109]

**Luis F. Fajardo L-G,** M.D.
Department of Pathology, Veterans Affairs Medical Center, Palo Alto, CA 94304 [7]

**Victor J. Ferrans,** M.D., Ph.D.
Pathology Branch, National Heart, Lung, and Blood Institute, National Institutes of Health, Bethesda, MD 20892 [25]

**Judy E. Garber,** M.D., M.P.H.
Division of Cancer Epidemiology and Control, Dana Farber Cancer Institute, Boston, MA 02115 [121]

**Joel W. Goldwein,** M.D.
Department of Radiation Oncology, Hospital of the University of Pennsylvania, Philadelphia, PA 19104-4283 [87,95]

**Daniel M. Green,** M.D.
Department of Pediatrics, Roswell Park Cancer Institute, Buffalo, NY 14263 [ix]

**Steven L. Hancock,** M.D.
Department of Radiation Oncology, Stanford University Medical Center, Stanford, CA 94305 [35]

**Gerd Hausdorf,** M.D., Ph.D.
Department of Congenital Heart Disease, German Heart Institute, D-1000 Berlin 65, Germany [73]

The numbers in brackets are the opening page numbers of the contributors' articles.

**Glenn Heller,** Ph.D.
Department of Pediatrics, Memorial Sloan-
Kettering Cancer Center, New York, NY
10021 [63]

**Eugene H. Herman,** Ph.D.
Division of Research and Testing, Food
and Drug Administration, Laurel, MD
20708 [25]

**Marc E. Horowitz,** M.D.
Pediatric Branch, National Cancer Institute,
National Institutes of Health, Bethesda,
MD 20892 [115]

**Regina I. Jakacki,** M.D.
Section of Pediatric Hematology/
Oncology, James Whitcomb Riley Hospital
for Children, Indianapolis, IN 46202-5225
[87,95]

**Ranae L. Larsen,** M.D.
Loma Linda University Medical Center,
Loma Linda CA [87,95]

**Steven E. Lipschultz,** M.D.
Department of Cardiology, Children's
Hospital, Boston, MA 02115 [45]

**Marilyn A. Masek,** B.A.
Department of Pathology, Stanford
University School of Medicine, Stanford,
CA 94305 [17]

**Linda McClure,** R.N.
Pediatric Branch, National Cancer Institute,
National Institutes of Health, Bethesda,
MD 20892 [115]

**David G. Poplack,** M.D.
Pediatric Branch, National Cancer Institute,
National Institutes of Health, Bethesda,
MD 20892 [115]

**Cindy L. Schwartz,** M.D.
Division of Pediatric Hematology-
Oncology, University of Rochester Medical
Center, Rochester, NY 14642 [103]

**Jeffrey H. Silber,** M.D., Ph.D.
Department of Pediatrics, Division of
Oncology, Children's Hospital of
Philadelphia, Philadelphia, PA 19104
[87,95]

**Laurel J. Steinherz,** M.D.
Department of Pediatrics, Memorial Sloan-
Kettering Cancer Center, New York, NY
10021 [63]

**Peter G. Steinherz,** M.D.
Department of Pediatrics, Memorial Sloan-
Kettering Cancer Center, New York, NY
10021 [63]

**Susie S. Truesdell,** P.A.
Division of Pediatric Cardiology,
University of Rochester Medical Center,
Rochester, NY 14642 [103]

# Preface

The therapy of children and adolescents with cancer has become increasingly successful, with over half of all those diagnosed now living five or more years after diagnosis. Most of these five-year survivors will never have a recurrence of the original cancer. As these survivors of childhood and adolescent cancer mature, they become aware of issues related to their original diagnosis and treatment of which they may have been unaware during the time of active therapy. These include quality-of-life issues, such as the availability of health and life insurance, educational and employment opportunities, and marriage and reproduction. Other concerns are survival expectancy and the possible occurrence of second malignant tumors.

The Second International Conference on the Long-Term Complications of Treatment of Children and Adolescents with Cancer was held in Buffalo, New York, from June 12th to 14th, 1992. The conference included fourteen invited presentations. Most of these concerned a single topic increasingly recognized as a potential cause of considerable excess mortality among survivors of childhood and adolescent cancer, i.e., treatment-related cardiac damage. The speakers discussed the pathology of radiation and anthracycline-related cardiac injury, the pathophysiology of anthracycline cardiomyopathy, the results of various strategies for screening survivors for the presence of treatment-related cardiomyopathy, and methods under development that may reduce the risk of anthracycline-related cardiac damage. The quality of the presentations was very high, with a lively interchange of data and opinions.

The focus of this volume is on the two agents most often implicated in cardiac damage, i.e., radiation therapy and anthracycline chemotherapy. Cyclophosphamide (CPM) is the only other agent in common use in pediatric oncology that has been associated with cardiac toxicity. Most, but not all, cases of fatal cardiac toxicity related to CPM have occurred in adults undergoing bone marrow transplantation, where there are several confounding variables in addition to that of patient age [1–3]. Even though this is a special problem applicable to a relatively small number of children, the reader should nonetheless be alert to this potentially devastating complication in transplant patients.

More relevant to pediatric oncology is the report by Makinen et al., who reported their studies of 35 long-term survivors of childhood cancer who had been followed for ten or more years after treatment with CPM [4]. Almost all had also received radiation therapy, other chemotherapeutic agents, or both modalities. Makinen et al. could not identify CPM as an independent risk factor for cardiac dysfunction, even though 24 of their patients had received 1000 mg/m²/week three or more times. They point out that even these high CPM doses are lower than those generally employed in preparative regiments for patients undergoing bone marrow transplantation.

There have been occasional individual reports of cardiac damage following treatment with combinations that have included dactinomycin, dacarbazine, 5-fluorouracil, and/or cisplatin. Most of these patients received other cardiotoxic therapies, so that the implicated drugs were, at most, co-factors [5-7].

This volume includes all the manuscripts prepared by the invited speakers to the conference. The diversity of opinion presented at the conference is reflected in the chapters of this book. It was clear from the speakers that we have much to learn regarding the optimal utilization and interpretation of the presently-available screening modalities. We have just begun to learn the natural history of radiation- and anthracycline-related cardiac injury. Dr. Garber's chapter reviews issues such as timing, disclosure of results, and intervention pertinent to presymptomatic screening, and relevant to cardiac as well as genetic screening.

The conference was co-sponsored by a generous educational grant from Adria Laboratories, Inc., and grants from the Association for Research of Childhood Cancer, Inc., Camp Good Days and Special Times, Inc., Roswell Park Cancer Institute, the National Cancer Institute, and the New York State Division, Inc., of the American Cancer Society.

The editors thank Mrs. Diane Piacente and Mrs. Rena Kaminski for typing the manuscripts.

## REFERENCES

1. Goldberg MA, Antin JH, Guinan EC, Rappaport JM: Cyclophosphamide cardiotoxicity: An analysis of dosing as a risk factor. Blood 68:1114–1118, 1986.
2. Mills BA, Roberts RW: Cyclophosphamide-induced cardiomyopathy. A report of two cases and review of the English literature. Cancer 43:2223–2226,1976.
3. Cazin B, Gorin NC, Laporte JP, Gallet B, Douay L, Lopez M, Najman A, Duhamel G: Cardiac complications after bone marrow transplantation. Cancer 57:2061–2069, 1986.
4. Makinen L, Makiperna A, Rautonen J, Heino M, Pyrhonen S, Laitinen LA, Siimes MA: Long-term cardiac sequelae after treatment of malignant tumors with radiotherapy or cytostatics in childhood. Cancer 65:1913–1917, 1990.
5. Kushner JR, Hansen VL, Hammar SP: Cardiomyopathy after widely separated courses of Adriamycin exacerbated by actinomycin D and mithramycin. Cancer 36:1577–1584, 1975.
6. Smith PJ, Ekert H, Waters KD, Matthews RN: High incidence of cardiomyopathy in children treated with Adriamycin and DTIC in combination chemotherapy. Cancer Treat Rep 61:1736–1738, 1977.
7. Jeremic B, Jevremovic S, Djuric L, Mijatovic L: Cardiotoxicity during chemotherapy with 5-fluorouracil and cisplatin. J Chemother 2:264–267, 1990.

**Daniel M. Green,** M.D.
**Giulio J. D'Angio,** M.D.
**J. Timothy Bricker,** M.D.

# 1. Perspectives Regarding Cardiac Complications of Cancer Therapy in Pediatric Patients

J. Timothy Bricker, M.D.

The discussions in this book provide a core of current knowledge essential for consultants in pediatric cardiology and pediatric oncology. Unfortunately, not all of the answers can be provided. Those seeking a simple recipe for patient management will be disappointed. A strategy that allows us to use anthracycline anticancer agents up to maximum effect but never beyond the point of danger is the Holy Grail that researchers in this field have been seeking.

The late onset of end-stage cardiac dysfunction as a sequel to therapy that saved the child's life is an overwhelming disaster in which the family and the child suffer twice. An equally terrible scenario is the child for whom the anthracyclines are the best (or perhaps even the only) chance for a cure, but because of an inordinately cautious approach to the prevention of late cardiac morbidity, the chance to cure is fatally compromised. The doctor caring for the child who has need of the anthracycline anticancer drugs must navigate the narrow channel between these two catastrophes, often with limited confidence in the estimations provided about how close the edge of danger might be. A number of different, sometimes conflicting, proposals have been put forth without adequate data for a consensus.

## MONITORING THE TOXICITY OF THERAPY

Better monitoring of cardiac toxicity and understanding of the long-term implications of minor or early cardiac abnormalities is an important area of research reflected in this volume. The optimal monitoring strategy in this regard would be a simple approach at low cost with an extremely high sensitivity for early changes predictive of late cardiac abnormality. Coupled with this would be a very low false-positive rate that would result in erroneous denial of anthracycline therapy. The diversity of approaches presented in this volume is a testimony to the fact that this optimal monitoring strategy has not yet been found.

The guidelines for monitoring, follow-up, and modification of therapy recommended by the Cardiology Committee of the Children's Cancer Group (in Steinherz et al., *Pediatrics* [1992] 89:942) were presented to provide more standardization of monitoring regimens, as well as with the intent to decrease the incidence of cardiac toxicity and to provide more comparable follow-up data for the evaluation of new protocols. Concern has been raised about the detection of subclinical findings that may not forecast an abnormality of functional importance and yet may precipitate

*Cardiac Toxicity After Treatment for Childhood Cancer*, pages 1–5, ©1993 Wiley-Liss, Inc.

decisions of profound consequence for the patient. Guidelines for therapy proposed by committees are found in situations in which the data are inadequate for a clear consensus based upon the data alone. Such guidelines stimulate research by those who are skeptical of the recommendations and, we hope, serve as a moving target as new data allow the modification of these guidelines.

There was a time when the clinician's guess regarding poor or good left ventricular function was based upon physical examination features such as the presence or absence of a gallop, crisp or muffled heart tones, heart enlargement by palpation or percussion, and so forth. It is easy to understand how cardiac enlargement from anemia or effusion could lead to a mistaken conclusion that the child had a dilated ventricle, or how severe hypovolemia in the setting of poor left ventricular wall movement could cause confusion. M-mode echocardiographic assessment of left ventricular chamber dimension and wall movement is an examination that provided a better estimate of the function of the left ventricle than did physical examination. While routine echocardiography does not measure ventricular contractility, clearly the patient with a greatly dilated left ventricle and very low degree of motion of the ventricular walls is likely to have a significant impairment of ventricular function. The M-mode left ventricular shortening fraction is a quick and convenient measurement that is easily communicated. This test has been followed closely by a number of centers with extensive pediatric chemotherapy experience over the years and bestows a visceral confidence that accompanies decisions about long-term follow-up. The problem in utilizing the M-mode shortening fraction to follow the asymptomatic child who needs anthracycline chemotherapy is that small increments of change in the percent shortening are very unlikely to reflect increments of change in ventricular function. Definite changes in shortening fraction can reflect a situation that is quite advanced and irreversible. The left ventricular shortening fraction by M-mode echocardiography is not totally worthless, but it is a measurement that is liable to be misinterpreted. Modest changes near the boundary between a "normal" and an "abnormal" percentage are apt to be due to changes in the filling conditions of the heart or the cardiac workload. There is enough subjectivity in determining where the endocardial surface begins to provide a variability in measurement of at least several percent, even when performed by the most diligent and particular echocardiographers.

In spite of the intuitive appeal of testing the cardiac reserve with exercise electrocardiogram (ECG)-gated nuclear cardiac blood pool (MUGA) scans, this test certainly does not provide a simple answer either. Normal children will have "abnormal" MUGA scans if normal adult responses are used for interpretation because failure of increase with exertion can be seen in normals. Abnormal resting left ventricular ejection fraction accompanied by symptoms of exercise intolerance can be associated with normalization of the left ventricular ejection fraction with exercise. By contrast, a fall in left ventricular ejection fraction with exercise can be associated with a normal cardiac index at peak exercise, as shown in Dr. Jakacki's data in this volume (Chapter 9). The practicality and costs of MUGA scans for routine follow-up have been questioned.

Electrocardiographic abnormalities are nonspecific. QT prolongation is found in many types of cardiomyopathy but has never been shown to be a sensitive or early sign. Screening strategies linked to electrocardiographic changes have not been found to have acceptable sensitivity or specificity in the past. The significance of ventricular arrhythmias is also unknown. There is no question that ventricular arrhythmia in the individual with impaired ventricular function is more ominous than in the setting of the child with a normal heart. However, the prediction of late events or late heart failure from premature ventricular contractions by Holter monitoring is limited by the small number of cases with long-term follow-up and sequential 24-hour electrocardiographic monitoring. The differences among centers may, in part, reflect differences in surveillance strategies.

Assessment of ventricular function in a manner that is relatively independent of the loading conditions of the heart has been a major contribution by Lipshultz and Colan to our diagnostic capabilities (see Chapter 6, this volume). The relationship between circumferential fiber shortening and end-systolic wall stress provides a very powerful index to address questions of contractility. The approach is certainly more involved than M-mode shortening fraction assessment. It can seem quite cumbersome on initial attempts, requires more specialized expertise, and takes a little additional time. However, it truly is feasible for this analysis to be provided on a routine basis by the echocardiographic laboratory of a children's hospital. It may be some time before load-free ventricular function testing is routinely available to all clinicians who follow children treated with anthracyclines. We nonetheless share the enthusiasm for this strategy for the assessment of ventricular function. This is especially true if one is intending to look for small or early changes in ventricular function near the range of normal cardiac performance on sequential follow-up studies. But availability of the stress–velocity index alone does not provide an answer to our need for a safe and simple outline for optimal use of anthracycline therapy without risk of cardiac toxicity. The long-term significance of minor changes in left ventricular function is not known. This long-lasting shortcoming of our cardiac assessment for this group of patients will be overcome by more precise and load-free measurements of ventricular contractility. Some patients who have cardiac dysfunction with thin-walled ventricles and with an abnormal afterload (from a structural cardiac standpoint) but with a normal arterial blood pressure and normal systemic vascular resistance may have normal contractility and a normal stress–velocity index. This concept may be novel to those who have been used to thinking of afterload in terms of blood pressure or vascular resistance. There are insufficient data to predict late heart complications with confidence based upon small (or even relatively large) changes in the stress–velocity index. Load-free contractility measurements will provide more interpretable documentation of small functional changes for future research applications of new protocols and for comparison of strategies for cardiac function preservation.

## REDUCING THE TOXICITY OF THERAPY

Another important area of research has emphasized approaches to optimize anti-cancer utility of these drugs while decreasing the probability of cardiac injury. The strategy of limiting dose has reduced late cardiac complications of anthracycline drug therapy. Limitations of this strategy include the fact that toxicity can occur late regardless of dose, that some tumors may need more than an arbitrary conservative maximum amount almost regardless of cardiac risk, and that the other contributors to risk in addition to the drug dosage cannot be accurately weighed. Dr.

Jakacki and coworkers provide evidence that being in a "low-risk" category by total dose of drug or radiation is not a guarantee of normal cardiac findings (see Chapter 9, this volume). There is no definite threshold that can be chosen to prevent risk totally and not inhibit salvage for some otherwise untreatable children. Nonetheless, the consensus is that this game plan has made the use of this class of drugs much safer from a cardiac standpoint.

Altering the infusion schedules to reduce the peak drug level has been advocated by Ewer and Benjamin to lower cardiac toxicity and provide a margin of safety in the setting in which tumor control becomes more crucial than the arbitrary total drug dosage (see Chapter 12, this volume). The work of Berg and associates is an extremely interesting approach to prevention of cardiac injury and holds great promise (Chapter 13, this volume).

The effect of intense cardiac physical training upon the cardiac function of the young person who has anthracycline administration is not known. As with most centers, we have former chemotherapy patients in the long-term follow-up program who are elite, intensely trained athletes. How beneficial or detrimental the effects of intense conditioning might be is unknown. When an exercise prescription and cardiac training are appropriate and when restriction from athletic participation should be recommended are decisions that must, as yet, be based upon personal biases and anecdotal observations.

## RECOMMENDATIONS

Drs. Lipshultz and Colan speculate about the $48 million annual economic impact of extensive monitoring of cardiac function (Chapter 6, this volume). Some might contest that the continuing cost of cardiac care for those suffering the lack of monitoring would be even higher than this, but it is impossible to prove or refute that allegation. What is clear is that a portion of a single-year cost of monitoring could certainly fund work to provide answers regarding the issues raised above. Prevention of anthracycline-related cardiac damage should be a prominent research priority.

Careful comparison of late cardiac outcome from centers with varying beliefs regarding treatment by pooling of data is difficult but might give insight into the value of dissimilar strategies. Great care would have to be given to similar assessment of normal or abnormal cardiac function if such a study were undertaken. Centers may also vary by the types of patients and thus the number who die before getting to the point of late cardiac complication. These are factors that should be taken into account in interpreting pooled data.

Variability in the vulnerability to cardiac complications adds to the difficulty of decisions in the individual case. The risks for development of anthracycline cardiotoxicity are only partly known. Total anthracycline dosage, age of the patient, gender, mediastinal irradiation, and ventricular function prior to drug treatment are contributors to the probability of a cardiac complication. Individual variations in myocardial activity of catalase, superoxide dismutase, and glutathione perioxidase might contribute to the risk. Microsomal coenzyme activities, unrecognized endogenous free radical scavengers, pretreatment iron status, selenium deficiency, and subclinical episodes of viral myocarditis could impart additional risk. It is possible that the risk factors for acute cardiac toxicity and chronic cardiac toxicity differ.

Mathematical modeling with multivariate analysis may provide additional information regarding some of these risk factors for future longitudinal studies. We are not able to use mathematical modeling and attribute anthracycline cardiotoxicity risk factors precisely to these variables for a number of reasons. Attempts to date to apply Bayesian analysis and multivariate modeling are laudable but have been limited by relatively small numbers of patients, arbitrary cutoff points in order to make categorical variables continuous variables, difficulty in identifying risks, and difficulty with endpoint determination.

Definitive cardiovascular endpoints such as cardiac mortality or severe cardiac disability initially seem easy to define in attempts to understand the contribution of various risk factors. Silber and coworkers emphasize that symptomatic cardiac limitations are important endpoints to consider with a potential for major impact upon the child's future (see Chapter 10, this volume). We are attempting to preserve cardiac reserve. Cardiac toxicity is a continuous rather than a categorical variable. However, we do not know how to predict loss of cardiac reserve or how much cardiac reserve will be enough. More proximate endpoints of cardiac damage (such as echocardiographic abnormalities or ventricular arrhythmias) are imperfect in predicting an eventual unfavorable outcome. Models with surrogate endpoints may or may not identify risk factors for cardiac complications. The information that compares one proximate endpoint with another rarely clarifies our understanding about risk factors for impending problems. It is not known whether "very late" complications will appear by their fourth or fifth decade for those children now determined to be free of cardiac complications using the long-term follow-up methods available to us at the present time.

Development of strategies to prevent or minimize cardiac toxicity while preserving the antineoplastic effect such as the project of Berg and associates (Chapter 13, this volume) are of utmost importance. In addition to the prevention of suffering, the cost-effectiveness of the success of this area of research will be recognizable, as emphasized by Lipshultz and Colan (Chapter 6, this volume). This must be highlighted as a priority for research funding.

How do we proceed as clinicians? Our strategy, for the present, continues to be fairly similar to that of the Cardiology Committee of the Children's Cancer Group guidelines cited above. Our team will look at the stress–velocity index periodically as well. Occasional cases with otherwise untreatable cancer will need to be given doses that exceed the guidelines. Safer infusion and scheduling strategies and the use of drugs to diminish toxicity will be carefully considered for our patients as more information becomes available.

The problem of judiciously navigating the misty narrow channel between cardiac toxicity and inappropriate limitations of treatment remains. Since we cannot clearly see either shore, we must attempt to steer as close to the center of the channel as possible while eagerly watching for the research funding that will allow the construction of better navigational equipment and the launch of a safer boat.

# 2. Pathology of Radiation-Induced Heart Disease

Luis F. Fajardo L-G, M.D.

Radiation-induced heart disease (RIHD) is the term coined in the late 1960s for the spectrum of clinical and pathological alterations of the heart occurring after therapeutic mediastinal irradiation [1,2]. Most RIHD patients have developed their disease after treatment for lymphomas (especially Hodgkin's disease); others were treated for tumors of the mediastinum such as thymomas, or for esophageal carcinoma, pulmonary and mammary neoplasms, etc. [1–4]. The morphologic alterations that occur in the heart and pericardium following exposure to ionizing radiation are closely dependent upon dose, irradiated volume, and time after exposure [4,5].

The clinical incidence of RIHD has varied in different series [4]. In our initial study of 318 patients at risk for at least 1 year following therapy for Hodgkin's disease, it was 6.6% overall [5]. In these series, each patient had 50% or more of the heart in the radiation field [5] and there was a well-defined dose response [5]. Of the few patients who had received doses of 5,500 cGy or more, 40% developed RIHD, and had the most severe lesions (e.g., combined pericardial and myocardial fibrosis) [5]. Other investigators have recorded a similar incidence [6]. However, some institutions have reported considerably higher figures [7,8], as much as 29% in one series [8]. Such high incidences may have resulted from different radiation techniques [4] or from different diagnostic criteria. In children and adolescents treated for Hodgkin's disease, both the risk and the severity of coronary heart disease appear to be higher (see below).

In our institution, since the mid-1970s the total dose to the heart has been limited by placing a subcarinal block after 3,000 cGy during therapy for lymphomas [9]. Since then the incidence of pericarditis has decreased to 2.5% [9].

Unfortunately, in the light of observations made within the last 10 years, it appears that long-term survivors of irradiated mediastinal neoplasms may have a high prevalence of subclinical functional abnormalities [10–13]. Although often asymptomatic, such patients may have low cardiac reserve and may not tolerate cardiovascular stress [10,14,15]. These patients may have pericardial thickening (up to 43% of them, by echocardiogram) [11]. However, the structural alterations that cause most of such minimal functional changes have eluded us, perhaps because they are within the wide spectrum of what we call "morphologically normal hearts."

The description of the pathology that follows refers generally to the changes of *clinically evident* RIHD, occurring after *therapeutic* irradiation. Injury to the heart can also occur in different circumstances, such as radiation accidents and atomic warfare, but these are not discussed here. As in many other tissues [16], the pathologic lesions produced by irradiation of the heart are not specific, but are characteristic enough to be recognized.

## ACUTE INJURY

It is quite likely that a transient acute granulocytic infiltrate occurs in the human heart hours after the initial doses of fractionated radiation to the mediastinum, and that it is generally asymptomatic and of little physiologic importance. This hypothesis is based on the sequential study of New Zealand White rabbits, which provide the best experimental model of RIHD [17]. However, for obvious reasons, it has not been proven histologically in humans so far.

In the rabbit model, 6 to 48 hours after single exposures of 1,800 to 2,000 cGy, there is extensive exudate of segmented granulocytes (heterophils in the rabbit) throughout all layers of the heart: parietal pericardium, epicardium, myocardium (around blood vessels), endocardium, and valves [17]. Neither fibrinous exudate nor structural alterations are detected by light microscopy and the cellular infiltrate disappears after 48 hours. Days after, damage to the myocardial capillary endothelium can be detected by electron microscopy [17,18]. As described below, the delayed lesions in the rabbit are identical to those of humans.

## DELAYED INJURY

The lesions described here are those appearing months to years after exposure and are the most important, clinically and morphologically. Each structure of the heart is considered separately.

## Parietal Pericardium

The parietal pericardium is by far the most frequently affected structure of the heart. There is fibrosis, characterized by dense collagen that replaces the outer, adipose layer. The thickness of the fibrous membrane is thereby increased from a normal of <1 mm (in the adult) to as much as >7 mm [3]. As in other organs, the collagen is haphazardly arranged in thick bundles [16]. Stromal fibrin can be detected, and there is practically always fibrinous exudate on the inner, mesothelial-lined surface that faces the heart [3,4]. Such fibrinous exudates may range from inconspicuous to massive, reaching occasionally the profuse amount and appearance observed in uremic pericarditis [4]. Although the vessels in such a fibrotic pericardium are prominent, very likely there is a reduction in the absolute number of blood capillaries, as compared with the normal; such a reduction has been demonstrated quantitatively in other irradiated tissues [18,19].

A modest exudate of lymphocytes, histiocytes, and plasma cells may be present near the surface; many cases, however, have no cellular exudate, in keeping with the characteristics of delayed radiation injury anywhere else [16]. Unless a neoplasm, infection, or trauma (e.g., surgical) is present, granulocytes are not seen at this late stage [3]. Pericardial fibrosis may progress to symptomatic constriction [20] in a proportion of cases (20% in one of our series) [21].

The mechanism of pericardial fibrosis has not been determined. As in other tissues such as skin or the alimentary tract, fibrosis might be the delayed result of ischemia. It is also quite possible that it may result from the organization (i.e., replacement by collagen) of long-standing fibrinous exudate. Fibrinous exudate is not only abundant (perhaps because the irradiated microvasculature is "leaky") but the normal resorption of fibrin is most likely impaired because of decrease in plasminogen activator, at least in endothelial cells [22]. Thus, collagen fibers eventually invade such long-standing fibrin deposits.

The pericardial lesion is almost always associated with exudate of protein-rich (up to 6 g of protein/dl) fluid in the pericardial sac. In fact, hydropericardium, symptomatic or not, may be the most common manifestation of RIHD; sometimes it may even be present without fibrosis. About one-half of the patients presenting with delayed pericardial disease had hydropericardium without clinical evidence of pericarditis, in one of our prospective studies [2]. The volume of this fluid varies from less than 50 ml to as much as 700 ml. Rapid accumulation of fluid can produce tamponade that occasionally proves to be lethal, particularly in patients who do not start with symptomatic pericarditis.

Pericardial disease, morphologically identical to that of humans, has been produced in New Zealand White rabbits by irradiating most of the heart with single doses (SD) of 1,800–2,000 cGy [5,17] or fractionated radiation (FR) of 5,400 cGy (12 equal fractions/28 days) [5,17]. The pericardial fibrosis and exudate occur 70 days or more after an SD. Their frequency and severity are clearly dose-dependent [5], as are those seen in humans [4,5]. Advanced lesions, with severe fibrosis and hydropericardium, lead to congestive failure and death [17]. In other animals (dogs, rats) radiation produces less pericardial fibrosis [23,24].

## Epicardium

The visceral pericardium is generally affected, although less frequently and severely than the parietal pericardium. Qualitatively the lesions are the same: fibrosis, fibrinous exudate, with little cellular inflammatory exudate.

Fibrous adhesions between epi- and pericardium are very rare, both in humans and in the rabbit model. In fact, the presence of extensive adhesions should suggest other causes instead of—or in addition to—radiation: tumor, trauma (such as surgery), infarcts, and infectious pericarditis should be considered. The cases of pericardial constriction, therefore, are not due to adhesions but to compression by a narrow pericardial sac.

## Myocardium

Less frequent than pericardial involvement, myocardial disease tends to be more severe and more often fatal. It may be isolated, but usually it is accompanied by pericardial fibrosis and exudate. The typical delayed lesion is diffuse myocardial fibrosis, in patches measuring from a few millimeters to several centimeters in maximum dimension, but never involving the entire myocardium [3,21]. We have seen those patches mostly in the anterior wall of the left ventricle; this may be related more to the geometry of the beam than to a particular susceptibility of this region.

The fibrosis consists of a network of mature collagen bundles (aniline blue positive), each usually having a width equal to, or less than, that of a myocyte [3,4,21]. The bundles surround individual myocytes or groups of myocytes, which otherwise do not appear abnormal. This fibrosis clearly replaces some myocytes, at the late (delayed) stage of the disease, but it is difficult to find necrotic or degenerating myocytes, and cellular inflammatory exudate is absent. These features distinguish delayed radiation-induced myocardial disease from other conditions also characterized by diffuse fibrosis, particularly myocarditis.

Radiation-induced diffuse fibrosis could occur in the conduction system and therefore lead to conduction defects of variable severity. However, instances of heart block or other arrhythmias are rare in our experience. In fact, many of those attributed by some observers to direct radiation effects on the conduction system could be explained by the far more common ischemia resulting from major coronary artery disease, whether radiation-induced or not.

Large scars of the type seen in myocardial infarcts are not seen unless there be severe coronary artery disease [1]. In such cases, the infarct has the same cause (acute ischemia), follows the usual physiopathologic sequence of events, and has the same morphology as ordinary myocardial infarcts [1,4] (see Coronary Arteries, below). Focal calcification of myocytes that presumably have undergone necrosis is seen occasionally, many years after exposure [4]. Probably such calcification is not extensive enough to interfere with myocardial function.

Rupture of the heart is an extraordinarily rare event, of which we know only of two instances in humans: a fatal ventricular perforation in a 48-year-old woman [25], and a right atriocutaneous fistula, in a 58-year-old woman, with intermittent bleeding that was surgically repaired [26]. It is not clear that radiation was the only cause—or even a cause—of such ruptures. We have never seen this complication in more than 500 rabbits irradiated with many multiple doses. However, in dogs, atrial necrosis and fistulae have been described [27–29].

The mechanism of diffuse myocardial fibrosis caused by radiation has been established in our laboratory using the rabbit model [18]. Following a single dose (SD) of 1,800 to 2,000 cGy, or comparable fractionated radiation (5,400 cGy in 12 FR/ 28 d), we have observed the sequential course of the disease, from a few minutes to >150 days [17,18]. An acute inflammatory exudate of granulocytes occurs in the myocardium and elsewhere in the heart between 6 and 48 hours after exposure. This exudate disappears in a few hours [17]. Progressive injury of endothelial cells in myocardial capillaries follows. It is detectable only by electron microscopy, and results in obstruction and/or destruction of capillaries. This reaches a maximum by 40 days post-SD exposure [18]. There is a transient endothelial cell proliferation detectable by $^3$HTdR autoradiography, but the myocardial microvasculature is compromised and the consequent ischemia results in progressive diffuse myocardial fibrosis. The type in humans is identical to that seen after single or fractionated dose radiation in rabbits; by analogy, the mechanism presumably is the same.

The initial acute inflammation in the rabbit model has been confirmed by other investigators [30]. The decrease in myocardial capillaries has also been confirmed in the rat, using different techniques (e.g., periodic acid–Schiff stain and injection of india ink [24,31]). In addition, researchers have studied the irradiated heart in different animal species: Such studies have focused on heart development (congenital anomalies and delay in growth after prenatal irradiation of rats) [32], metabolic alterations (decrease in ATP and transport-ATPase as well as noradrenaline in guinea pigs [33]), dose response for pericardial disease in dogs (lower threshold than in rabbits) [23], coronary artery disease in rabbits (see below), cardiac function [34], decrease in cardiac output in rats [35,36], conduction defects (junctional and atrial tachycardias, atrial fibrillation, atrioventricular block in dogs, following high doses) [29], and enzyme profiles in the myocardium (decreased alkaline phosphatase and 5'-nucleotidase in rat myocardial capillaries) [31,36].

## Parietal Endocardium

Focal fibrous thickening may occur in the left ventricular endocardium, with proliferation of elastic fibers [3,4]. This fibroelastosis appearing in cushionlike areas is probably of little physiologic importance.

In $C_3H$ mice, we have consistently produced an extensive mural thrombosis of the ventricles whose incidence and severity are dose-dependent (SD of 1,200 to 4,000 cGy) [37]. The thrombus is eventually replaced by collagen and it does not affect survival in animals followed up to 6 months [37]. Since this thrombosis implies injury of the endocardial endothelium, and since there is no myocardial fibrosis, the evidence suggests that, at least in this mouse strain, the endothelial cells of the endocardium are more radiosensitive than those of the myocardial capillaries. Exactly the opposite occurs in the rabbit and probably in humans.

## Valves

Thickening of the valvular endocardium has been described in some necropsies of young adults [38]. Also, some cases of valvular disease have been described *clinically* [1,7,39]. The causal role of radiation has never been clearly established, however, and other possible etiologies cannot be ruled out. We have not found in our series any instances of valvular disease in humans that can be unquestionably attributed to radiation [4]. Moreover, in the several hundred rabbits irradiated at various dose levels, we have not observed any valvular lesions [4,17].

In fact, there is no reason to expect valvular disease after radiation. Most delayed radiation effects are mediated through *vascular damage* [16] and the heart valves *do not contain blood vessels*. There is no evidence that the endothelium that covers the valves is particularly sensitive to radiation. Nevertheless, we cannot rule out completely the possibility that radiation-induced valvular disease may occur in extremely rare instances.

## Coronary Arteries

Coronary artery disease (CAD) caused or aggravated by radiation has been considered uncommon until recently [40] for good reasons. The morphology of arterial lesions caused by radiation is essentially the same as that produced by spontaneous atherosclerosis. Therefore radiation can only be blamed for CAD in patients who are too young to have spontaneous atherosclerosis or in those whose coronary arterial lesions in the irradiated field are clearly more severe than those of nonirradiated arteries of similar caliber. Within those caveats only a few of the cases claimed up to the late 1980's appeared to be truly radiation-induced CAD, although the number of reports had been increasing steadily in the last decade [39–45].

In recent months several studies have indicated that CAD is indeed an important late manifestation of cardiac irradiation [44,45a,45b]. A recent study of patients treated for Hodgkin's disease and followed for an average of 7 years indicates an overall relative risk for death with coronary artery disease of 1.87 and for myocardial infarct of 2.56 [44]. This study is based on death certificates and therefore is not as objective as those based on actual necropsy findings. It nevertheless does indicate an increased risk for CAD [44]. An excess mortality due to CAD was also observed in Scandinavian women treated by high-dose radiation for breast cancer, as compared with those treated by surgery alone [45a].

The most compelling observation is one published in this volume (Chapter 5). The authors reviewed 635 patients irradiated at Stanford for Hodgkin's disease before age 21, in the years 1961 to 1991. The relative risk of death from myocardial infarction (as compared to controls matched for age, sex, and race) was 41.5 (confidence intervals of 18.1 to 82.1) [45b]. If these and similar observations are accurate predictors, we should see a significant rise in radiation-associated coronary artery disease, especially among patients treated during childhood.

Some investigators have been skeptical about the association of radiation and CAD [40,45], especially with current radiotherapy techniques [40,46]. Other researchers wisely suggest that more experience is necessary before therapeutic radiation can be considered *a major cause* of CAD [39,47].

The lesions of radiation-associated CAD are those of arterio- and atherosclerosis: intimal proliferation containing collagen, myofibroblasts, macrophages, lipids, cholesterol, and fibrin, and causing concentric or eccentric reduction of the vascular lumen, with or without thrombosis [1,3]. The resulting ischemic effects are no different from those of spontaneous atherosclerosis: angina pectoris, myocardial infarct, and sudden death [1,40,45,46].

Radiation alone cannot produce coronary atherosclerosis in experimental animals; the addition of a high-lipid diet is necessary unless the animal already has hyperlipidemia [45,48]. The latter, of course, is often present in humans. Therefore, radiation should not be viewed as an *independent* cause of CAD, but as a cofactor.

## ANTHRACYCLINE CARDIO-TOXICITY AND RADIATION

It has been suggested that antineoplastic chemotherapy compounds known to be cardiotoxic can potentiate—or be potentiated by—radiation [12,42,49,50].

An interaction between radiation and chemotherapy has been demonstrated well in the case of the anthracyclines [51–53]. Adriamycin (doxorubicin) has been recognized as a cardiotoxic compound for many years [54]. It often produces a cardiomyopathy, which is dose-dependent [55,56].

Morphologically it is characterized by myocyte damage: There is dilatation of the sarcotubular system and loss of myofibrils, with fragmentation of myofilaments, which initially can only be detected at the ultrastructural level [37,38]. Cells totally devoid of contractile elements can remain for some time and be recognized as characteristic basophilic elements ("Adria cells"), which are otherwise not specific [51,57,58]. This random damage of myocytes is best diagnosed and graded by electron microscopy. Several endomyocardial biopsies should be examined when making a decision about further Adriamycin therapy, especially in patients who have already received $\geq 450$ mg/m$^2$, or who are in the risk categories for anthracycline cardiotoxicity [50]. Such risk factors include pre-existing heart disease (valvular, coronary, myocardial), hypertension, age >70 years, and prior mediastinal irradiation [50].

The ultimate effect of Adriamycin cardiotoxicity is diffuse myocardial fibrosis, as demonstrated in the rabbit [57,58], which is not only a good model for radiation injury but also for anthracycline cardiomyopathy. In humans, however, heart failure often occurs before extensive fibrosis develops, while in rabbits diffuse fibrosis is well advanced at the time of failure. Diffuse myocardial fibrosis can therefore be considered a common endpoint in both radiation and Adriamycin cardiomyopathy [58], but the pathway to fibrosis is different for each. In radiation, it occurs through endothelial damage, causing microvascular deficit and resulting in ischemia [18]. The damage with Adriamycin occurs in myocytes that are eventually replaced by fibrous tissue [58].

As indicated above, Adriamycin does aggravate radiation injury in the myocardium. Clinical evidence suggested that the interaction was synergistic [51,59], but a large, unique experiment using several hundred rabbits proved that the effects are additive rather than synergistic, at least at low and moderate doses of the anthracycline [52,60]. Regardless of the mode of interaction, it is clear that the use of cardiac radiation and Adriamycin (sequentially or concomitantly) increases the patient's risk for the development of cardiac disease following doses of each agent ordinarily considered safe [4,60].

## REFERENCES

1. Cohn KE, Stewart JR, Fajardo LF, Hancock W: Heart disease following radiation. Medicine 46:281–298, 1967.
2. Stewart JR, Cohn KE, Fajardo LF, Hancock W, Kaplan HS: Radiation-induced heart disease. A study of twenty-five patients. Radiology 89:302–310, 1967.
3. Fajardo LF, Stewart JR, Cohn KE: Morphology of radiation-induced heart disease. ArchPathol86: 512–519, 1986.
4. Stewart JR, Fajardo LF: Radiation-induced heart disease: An update. Prog Cardiovasc Dis 27:173–194, 1984.
5. Stewart JR, Fajardo LF: Dose response in human and experimental radiation-induced heart disease. Application of the nominal standard dose (NSD) concept. Radiology 99:403–408, 1971.
6. Kurichety PR, Mill WB, Prasad SC, Lee J: Radiation-induced pericarditis in mantle irradiation: An analysis of causative factors. Int J Radiat Oncol Biol Phys 6:1366–1367, 1980 (abstr).
7. Morton DL, Glancy DL, Joseph WL, Adkins PC: Management of patients with radiation-induced pericarditis with effusion: A note on the development of aortic regurgitation in two of them. Chest 64:291–297, 1973.
8. Byhardt R, Brace K, Ruckdeschel J, Chang P, Martin R, Wiernik P: Dose and treatment factors in radiation-related pericardial effusion associated with the mantle technique for Hodgkin's disease. Cancer 35:795–802, 1975.
9. Carmel RJ, Kaplan HS: Mantle irradiation in Hodgkin's disease. Cancer 37:2813–2825, 1976.
10. Gottdeiner JS, Katin MJ, Borer JS, Bachrach SL, Green MV: Late cardiac effects of therapeutic mediastinal irradiation: Assessment by echocardiography and radionuclide angiography. N Engl J Med 308:569–572, 1983.
11. Green DM, Gingell RL, Pearce J, Panahon AM, Ghoorah J: The effects of mediastinal irradiation on cardiac function of patients treated during childhood and adolescence for Hodgkin's disease. J Clin Oncol 5:239–245, 1987.
12. Makinen L, Makipernaa A, Rautonen J, Heino M, Pyrhonen S, Laitinen LA, Siimes MA: Long-term cardiac sequelae after treatment of malignant tumors with radiotherapy or cytostatics in childhood. Cancer 65:1913–1917, 1990.
13. Savage DE, Constine LS, Schwartz RG, Rubin P: Radiation effects on left ventricular function and myocardial perfusion in long term survivors of Hodgkin's disease. Int J Radiat Oncol Biol Phys 19:721–727, 1990.
14. Morgan GW, Freeman AP, McLean RG, Jarvie BH, Giles RW: Late cardiac, thyroid and pulmonary sequelae of mantle radiotherapy for Hodgkin's disease. Int J Radiat Oncol Biol Phys 11:1925–1931, 1985.
15. Watchie J, Coleman CN, Raffin TA, Cox R, Raubitscheck A, Fahey T, Hoppe R, Van Kessel A: Minimal long-term cardio-pulmonary dysfunction following treatment for Hodgkin's disease. Int J Radiat Oncol Biol Phys 13:517–524, 1987.
16. Fajardo LF (ed): Pathology of Radiation Injury. New York: Masson Publishing, USA, 1982.
17. Fajardo LF, Stewart JR: Experimental radiation-induced heart disease. I. Light microscopic studies. Am J Pathol 59:299–316, 1970.
18. Fajardo LF, Stewart JR: Pathogenesis of radiation-induced myocardial fibrosis. Lab Invest 29:244–257, 1973.
19. Archambeau J, Ines A, Fajardo LF: Response of swine skin microvasculature to acute single exposures of x-rays: Quantification of endothelial changes. Radiat Res 98:37–51, 1984.
20. Greenwood RD, Rosenthal A, Cassady R, Jaffe N, Nadas AS: Constrictive pericarditis in childhood due to mediastinal irradiation. Circulation 50:1033–1039, 1974.
21. Fajardo LF, Stewart JR: Radiation-induced heart disease. Human and experimental observations. In MR Bristow (ed): Drug-Induced Heart Disease. Amsterdam: Elsevier, North-Holland Bio-

medical Press, 1980, pp 241–260.

22. Fajardo LF: The unique physiology of endothelial cells and its implications in radiobiology. Front Radiat Ther Oncol 23:96–112, 1989.

23. Gavin PR, Gillette EL: Radiation response of the canine cardiovascular system. Radiat Res 90:489–500, 1982.

24. Lauk S, Kiszel Z, Buschmann J, Trott KR: Radiation-induced heart disease in rats. Int J Radiat Oncol Biol Phys 11:801–808, 1985.

25. Rubin E, Camara J, Grayzel DM, Zak FG: Radiation-induced cardiac fibrosis. Am J Med 34:71–75, 1963.

26. Conklin EF, Whalen WP, Rose M, Gianelli Jr S: Cutaneous fistula of right atrium following irradiation. NY State J Med 74(9):1643–1644, 1974.

27. Stryker JA, Lee KJ, Abt AB: The effects of X radiation on the canine heart. Radiat Res 82:200–210, 1980.

28. Zook BC, Bradley EW, Casarett GW, Rogers CC: Pathologic changes in the hearts of beagles irradiated with fractionated fast neutrons or photons. Radiat Res 88:607–618, 1981.

29. Dick HLH, Saylor CB, Reeves MM, Davies MJ: Chronic cardiac arrhythmias produced by focused Cobalt-60 gamma irradiation of the canine atria. Radiat Res 78:390–403, 1979.

30. Maeda S: Pathology of experimental radiation pancarditis. I. Observation on radiation-induced heart injuries following a single dose of x-ray irradiation to rabbit heart with special reference to its pathogenesis. Acta Pathol Jpn 30:59–78, 1980.

31. Lauk S, Trott KR: Endothelial cell proliferation in the rat heart following local heart irradiation. Int J Radiat Biol 567:1017–1030, 1990.

32. Martin PG: Postnatal growth in prenatally irradiated rats: II. Exposure rate effects of the adrenal, pituitary, lung, heart and testes. Growth 37:165–175, 1973.

33. Prignitz R, Saurbier B, Hoffmeister G: Untersuchungen uber den Einfluss von Rontgenstrahlen auf Elektrolytverschiebungen und Stoffwechsel des Herzmuskels. VI. Strahlenbedingte Veranderungen des Katecholamingehaltes. Strahlentherapie 151:53–60, 1976.

34. Keyeux A: Functional response of heart and major vessels. Curr Topics Radiat Res Quarterly 10:98–108, 1974.

35. Yeung TK, Hopewell JW: Effects of single doses of radiation on cardiac function in the rat. Radiother Oncol 3:339–345, 1985.

36. Yeung TK, Lauk S, Simmonds RH, Hopewell JW, Trott KR: Morphological and functional changes in the rat heart after x-irradiation: Strain differences. Radiat Res 119:489–499, 1989.

37. Brown JM, Fajardo LF, Stewart JR: Mural thrombosis of the heart induced by radiation. Arch Pathol 96:1–4, 1973.

38. Brosius FC, Waller BF, Roberts WG: Radiation heart disease: Analysis of 16 young (aged 15 to 33 years) necropsy patients who received over 3500 rads to the heart. Am J Med 70:519–530, 1981.

39. Hancock SL, Hoppe RT, Horning SJ, Rosenberg SA: Intercurrent death after Hodgkin's disease therapy in radiotherapy and adjuvant MOPP trials. Ann Intern Med 109:183–189, 1988.

40. Stewart JR, Fajardo LF: Cancer and coronary artery disease (editorial). Int J Radiat Oncol Biol Phys 4:915–916, 1978.

41. Joensuu H: Acute myocardial infarction after heart irradiation in young patients with Hodgkin's disease. Chest 95:388–390, 1989.

42. Trigg ME, Finlay JL, Boxdech M, Gilbert E: Fatal cardiac toxicity in bone marrow transplant patients receiving cytosine arabinoside, cyclophosphamide and total body irradiation. Cancer 59:38–42, 1987.

43. Pohjla-Sintonen S, Totterman KJ, Salmo M, Siltanen P: Late cardiac effects of mediastinal radiotherapy in patients with Hodgkin's disease. Cancer 60:31–37, 1987.

44. Boivin JF, Hutchison GB, Lubin JH, Mauch P: Coronary artery disease mortality in patients treated for Hodgkin's disease. Cancer 69:1241–1247, 1992.

45. Fajardo LF: Radiation-induced coronary artery disease (editorial). Chest 71:563–564, 1977.

45a. Rutquist LE, Lax I, Fornander T, Johansson H: Cardiovascular mortality in a randomized trial of adjuvant radiation therapy versus surgery alone in primary breast cancer. Int J Radiat Oncol Biol Phys 22:887–896, 1992.

45b. Hancock SL, Donaldson SS: Radiation-related heart disease: Risks after treatment of Hodgkin's disease during childhood and adolescence. This volume, Chapter 5, pp. 35–43.

46. Corn BW, Trock BJ, Goodman R: Irradiation-related ischemic heart disease. J Clin Oncol 8:741–750, 1990.

47. Lederman GS, Sheldon TA, Chaffey JT, Herman TS, Gelman RS, Coleman CN: Cardiac disease after mediastinal irradiation for seminoma. Cancer 60:772–776, 1987.

48. Amromin GD, Gildenhorn HL, Soloman RD, Nadkarni BB, Jacobs ML: The synergism of x-irradiation and cholesterol-fat feeding on the development of coronary artery lesions. J Atherosclerosis Res 4:325–334, 1964.

49. Phillips TL, Fu KK: The interaction of drug and radiation effects on normal tissues. Int J Radiat Oncol Biol Phys 4:59–64, 1978.

50. Bristow MR (ed): Anthracycline cardiotoxicity.

In Drug-Induced Heart Disease. Amsterdam: Elsevier/North Holland, 1980, pp 191–215.

51. Billingham ME, Bristow MR, Glatstein E, Mason JW, Masek MA, Daniels JR: Adriamycin cardiotoxicity. Endomyocardial biopsy evidence of enhancement of irradiation. Am J Surg Pathol 1:17–23, 1977.

52. Eltringham JR, Fajardo LF, Stewart JR: Adriamycin cardiomyopathy: Enhanced cardiac damage in rabbits with combined drug and cardiac irradiation. Radiology 115:471–472, 1975.

53. Belli JA, Piro AJ: The interaction between radiation and Adriamycin damage in mammalian cells. Cancer Res 37:1624–1630, 1977.

54. Lefrak EA, Pitha J, Rosenheim S, Gottleib JA: A clinico-pathologic analysis of Adriamycin cardiotoxicity. Cancer 32:302–314, 1973.

55. Gilladoga AC, Tan CT, Phillips FSS, Sternberg S, Tang CK, Wollner N, Murphy ML: Cardiac status of 40 children receiving Adriamycin over

495 mg/m² and animal studies. Proc Am Assoc Cancer Res 15:107, 1974 (abstr).

56. Minow RA, Benjamin RS, Lee ET, Gottlieb JA: Adriamycin cardiomyopathy—risk factors. Cancer 39:1397–1401, 1977.

57. Jaenke R, Fajardo LF: Summary report on Adriamycin-induced myocardial lesions. Report of a workshop. Am J Surg Pathol 1:55–60, 1977.

58. Fajardo LF, Eltringham JR, Stewart JR: Combined cardiotoxicity of Adriamycin and x-radiation. Lab Invest 34:86–96, 1976.

59. Merrill J, Greco FA, Zimbler H, Brereton HD, Lamberg JD, Pomeroy TC: Adriamycin and radiation: Synergistic cardiotoxicity. Ann Intern Med 82:122, 1975.

60. Eltringham JR, Fajardo LF, Stewart JR, Klauber MR: Investigation of cardiotoxicity in rabbits from Adriamcyin and fractionated cardiac irradiation: Preliminary results. Front Radiat Ther Oncol 13:21–35, 1979.

# 3. The Pathology of Anthracycline Cardiotoxicity in Children, Adolescents, and Adults

Margaret E. Billingham, M.B., B.S., F.R.C. Path., and Marilyn A. Masek, B.A.

The anthracycline antibiotics are useful chemotherapeutic agents when used alone or in combination chemotherapy. Since the introduction of doxorubicin into clinical use in the early 1970s [1], it has been known that cardiotoxicity was the limiting factor in the usefulness of this drug and other anthracycline analogs [2]. It is also well known that the cardiotoxic effects of anthracyclines are dose related, and the incidence of heart failure is less if the cumulative dose of doxorubicin is limited to less than 500 mg/m$^2$, whereas the incidence climbs in patients receiving a greater total dose [3]. It is also known, however, that there is considerable variation in the tolerance to doxorubicin between patients, and that certain risk factors, such as radiation to the mediastinum, old age, and other cardiac diseases, may cause the development of cardiotoxicity at a cumulative dose of less than 500 mg/m$^2$ [3]. The use of endomyocardial biopsy for grading cardiac histology is now accepted as a means of predicting cardiotoxicity in certain larger centers, particularly the M.D. Anderson Hospital (Houston) and Stanford University Medical Center. The morphologic signs of cardiotoxicity have been described previously, as has the use of the grading to predict and monitor anthracycline cardiotoxicity [4–6]. Endomyocardial bi-

opsy has been employed less frequently to monitor children receiving anthracyclines. The purpose of this chapter is to review the morphologic changes of anthracycline cardiotoxicity in the adult and to compare these changes with those found in children and adolescents. A National Cancer Institute study showed that more than half of the patients treated with doxorubicin developed drug-induced cardiotoxicity [7]. At this time, none of the new anthracycline analogs have shown a clear advantage over the original compounds. It is hoped that new analogs will be found that will have less cardiotoxicity without loss of antitumor activity.

## METHODS

### Patients

This study describes the morphologic changes of patients who had been treated with the anthracycline antibiotics in varying doses for various tumor types. In the study, the patients were divided into three groups (Table 1): Group A: A total of 867 biopsies were studied in patients ranging from 9 months to 82 years (with a mean of 47.8 years); 486 were female and 339 were male (in 42 cases the sex was not known). Group B consisted of 76 endomyocardial

**TABLE 1.  Age Range and Sex of Patients Studied for Anthracycline Cardiotoxicity**

| Group | Biopsy Nos. | Age Range | Sex |
|-------|-------------|-----------|-----|
|       |             |           | F:M |
| A     | 867         | 9 mo–82 yr (mean 47.8 yr) | 486:339[a] |
| B     | 76          | 9 mo–20 yr (mean 12.9 yr) | 27:38[b] |
| C     | 35          | 9 mo–15 yr (mean 8.13 yr) | 5:10 |

[a]In 42 cases, sex not known.
[b]In 11 cases, sex not known.

biopsies in anthracycline-treated patients ranging in age from 9 months to 20 years (with a mean of 12.9 years), of which 27 were female and 38 were male (in 11 cases, the sex was unknown). The third group, group C, consisted of 35 endomyocardial biopsies in anthracycline-treated children ranging in age from 9 months to 15 years (with a mean of 8.13 years), in which 5 were female and 10 were male. All the patients being treated had tumors of various types in groups B and C. The tumors included Wilms' tumor, neuroblastoma, Ewing's sarcoma, osteosarcoma, malignant histiocytosis, and Burkitt's and other lymphomas. All of the patients had endomyocardial biopsies with a range of cardiotoxicity varying from grades 1 to 3. The majority of patients were treated with doxorubicin. However, some were treated with daunomycin, dioxydoxorubicin, and 4'-epirubicin. Two other patients were included in the study who had no endomyocardial biopsies, but who died as a result of acute doxorubicin cardiotoxicity (pericarditis–myocarditis syndrome), and the autopsied heart pathology is briefly described.

## Electron Microscopy

Tissue obtained by endomyocardial biopsy consisted of enough tissue to make 10 epon blocks (at least three pieces of myocardium from different areas of the right ventricular septum). The tissue was fixed in 2.5% glutaraldehyde with 2% paraformaldehyde in 0.1 M sodium cacodylate buffer (pH 7.2) for electron microscopy. Sections of epon plastic-embedded myocardium 1-micron-thick were screened by light microscopy for overall assessment and the three blocks showing the most severe changes were then screened by electron microscopy for grading.

## Endomyocardial Biopsy

All of the biopsies of this study were obtained by endomyocardial biopsy. The technique for this procedure has been well-described previously [8]. The type and size of the bioptome used varied with adults and children. In most cases, the adults' biopsies were obtained with a 9 French bioptome (Stanford), although sometimes the Cordis 7 French bioptome was used. For children and infants, the sizes of the bioptomes used were much smaller. Briefly, the endomyocardial bioptome is placed percutaneously over a guide wire in the right internal jugular vein using the Seldinger technique. The bioptome is passed into the right ventricle, where the biopsy is obtained. The tissue obtained is fixed immediately. This technique can be performed on an outpatient basis.

## RESULTS

There were no deaths or serious morbidity as a result of the endomyocardial biopsies described in this study. The endomyocardial biopsy yielded good tissue for ultrastructural studies (Fig. 1). The pathologic changes seen by ultrastructure showed two types of lesions in the myocytes. The lesions were focal, some-times one affected myocyte surrounded by normal myocardium. At other times, clusters of myocytes or all myocytes were affected. Two main types of myocyte injury were seen ultrastructurally in anthra-

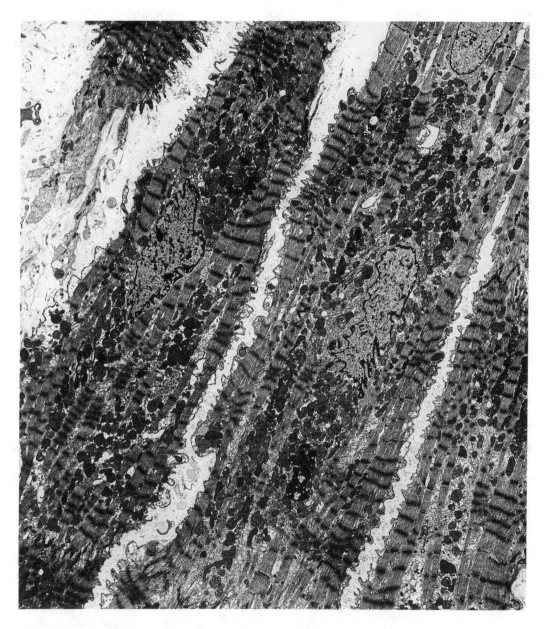

**Fig. 1.** Electron micrograph showing unaffected myocardium from a 10-year-old child. ×4,320.

cycline cardiotoxicity: The first was myofibrillar loss within individual myocytes. Initially, the cell may be only partialy affected, but then the whole cell shows myofibrillar loss, with only Z-band remnants remaining around the cell margin (Fig. 2). The nuclei appear unaffected and are not enlarged. The mitrochondria are seen to contain compact cristae, although they were often smaller than in the surrounding unaffected myocytes. The myocytes with total myofibrillar loss were easily recognized on thick plastic sections. As in animal and human studies, previously described [4], the second type of myocyte injury showed vacuolar degeneration and coalescence of the swollen sarcotubular system (Fig. 2). These changes also occur with preservation of the nucleus and the mitochondria. These two types of myocyte-degenerative change seen in anthracycline cardiotoxicity are sometimes seen one at a time in any biopsy, or both types of change may be seen in the same biopsy (Fig. 2). In our experience, the myofibrillar loss is more common than the vacuolar degeneration in humans. There does not seem to be a relationship between the two types of injury and the severity of cardiotoxicity. There is nearly always an increase in interstitial fibrosis in anthracycline cardiotoxicity. If the grade of toxicity is high, necrotic myocytes are seen. Inflammatory infiltrates and vasculitis are not a feature of chronic anthracycline cardiotoxicity. Patients treated with anthracycline analogs of doxorubicin—DNA, daunomycin, AD-32, Rubidazine, Carminomycin, and 4'-epirubicin—all show similar morphologic changes, with both types of cell damage described above, although these may occur at different cumulative doses.

In order to make more meaningful clinicopathologic correlations and quantitative estimates, it is necessary to have a grading system to quantitate the morphological changes. The grading systems have been described in previous publications [6], and the grading system used is shown in Table 2. Both types of myocyte damage are graded equally. Before grading anthracycline cardiotoxicity, there must be at least 10 blocks of tissue. Otherwise a numerical value should not be given. The pitfalls include mistaking lipid droplets within the myocyte for swollen sarcotubular reticulum. Myofibrillar loss should only be called when Z-band remnants can be seen around the periphery of the cell. Fibrosis, although present in anthracycline cardiotoxicity, is not considered in the grading system because it may result from nonspecific changes or may be due to previous radiation effect. Although severe cardiotoxic changes can be detected by conventional microscopy, it is preferable to use 1-micron-thick plastic sections and electron microscopy to grade these cellular changes accurately. Our study shows

**TABLE 2.  Morphologic Grading System for Cardiotoxicity**

| Grade | Morphology |
| --- | --- |
| 0 | Normal myocardial ultrastructural morphology |
| 1 | Isolated myocytes affected by distended sarcotubular system and/or early myofibrillar loss; damage to <5% of all cells in 10 plastic blocks |
| 1.5 | Changes similar to those in grade 1, but with damage to 6–15% of all cells in 10 plastic blocks. |
| 2.0 | Clusters of myocytes affected by myofibrillar loss and/or vacuolization, with damage to 16–25% of all cells in 10 plastic blocks. |
| 2.5[a] | Many myocytes, 26–35% of all cells in 10 plastic blocks, affected by vacuolization and/or myofibrillar loss. |
| 3.0[a] | Severe and diffuse myocyte damage (>35% of all cells in 10 plastic blocks) affected by vacuolization and/or myofibrillar loss. |

[a]At grade 2.5, only one more dose of anthracycline should be given without further evaluation. At grade 3.0, no more anthracycline should be given.

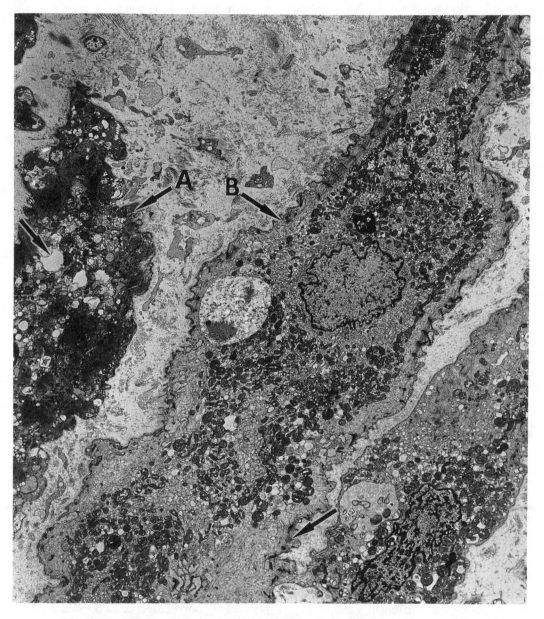

**Fig. 2.** Electron micrograph showing myocardium from a 10-year-old child with grade 3 anthracycline cardiotoxicity. Note myofibrillar loss with peripheral Z-band remnants (arrow) in myocyte B and sarcotubular swelling (arrow) in myocyte A. ×4,320.

that anthracycline-associated myocardial degeneration occurred in virtually all patients treated with doses in excess of 240 mg/m$^2$. The lowest dose at which anthracycline-related change was seen was 180 mg/m$^2$. As has been shown previously, radiation enhances anthracycline cardiotoxicity either before or after anthracycline administration [9,10]. This is true also for some of the anthracycline analogs. In some cases, anthracycline may induce a "recall" phenomenon of acute radiation change in the myocardial small vessels. Although the morphologic ultrastructural changes of anthracycline administration described here are quite characteristic of anthracycline damage, they are not entirely specific, and similar changes are sometimes seen in end-stage idiopathic dilated cardiomyopathies. There are, however, morphometric ways to distinguish the changes in cardiomyopathies from anthracycline cardiotoxicity [11].

In the case of the two adults who died from presumed "acute anthracycline cardiotoxicity" within days of receiving doxorubicin, the hearts both showed a fibrinous pericarditis with adjacent myocarditis of predominantly lymphocytes.

## Morphological Changes in Children and Adolescents

In this study, 76 biopsies were from patients aged from 9 months to 20 years with a mean of 12.9 years. There were no deaths or morbidity due to the endomyocardial biopsy in this group. The morphologic changes described for anthracycline cardiotoxicity were identical to those described above for adults. In group C, the only other change noted, apart from those described above for adults, was the more frequent appearance of lipid droplets within myocytes that could easily be distinguished from swelling of the sarcotubular reticulum (Fig. 3) in children under 10 years. The presence of lipid does not preclude an accurate grading of the endomyocardial biopsies.

The morphologic grading system, sometimes together with right heart catheterization, was used throughout to manage the patients in these studies.

## DISCUSSION

Endomyocardial biopsy has made possible early morphologic detection of anthracycline cardiotoxicity in adults and children. The evolution of cardiotoxicity and its clinicopathologic correlations have been elucidated with this morphologic grading. These advances have now been extended to the pediatric age group, even infants, in whom endomyocardial biopsy can now be performed. A recent study by Yoshizato et al. described the result of 66 endomyocardial biopsy procedures in 53 children with a mean age of 13 years [12]. The question of morbidity of endomyocardial biopsy in children is important. It should be remembered that infants and very young children sometimes require general anesthesia to obviate the possibility of air embolus occurring while they are crying during the procedure. Serious complications in children, however, are rare in other reported series, although, in the study referred to above, three cardiac perforations were recorded. None of them was fatal. This higher rate of perforation might have been due to the exclusive use of the femoral approach by this group. It should be obvious, however, that endomyocardial biopsy in very young children should be performed only by skilled and experienced invasive cardiologists or surgeons.

The endomyocardial biopsy score has been shown to have a predictive value. The data in consecutive biopsies in any one patient consistently show a linear relationship between the biopsy score and anthracycline dose for group or individual data. It is therefore predictive of the degree of toxicity even at an early stage of drug administration [13]. In contrast, functional tests (hemodynamic, electrophysiologic, and echocardiographic) show little or no cardiac function abnormality at low doses of the drug, even when serial stud-

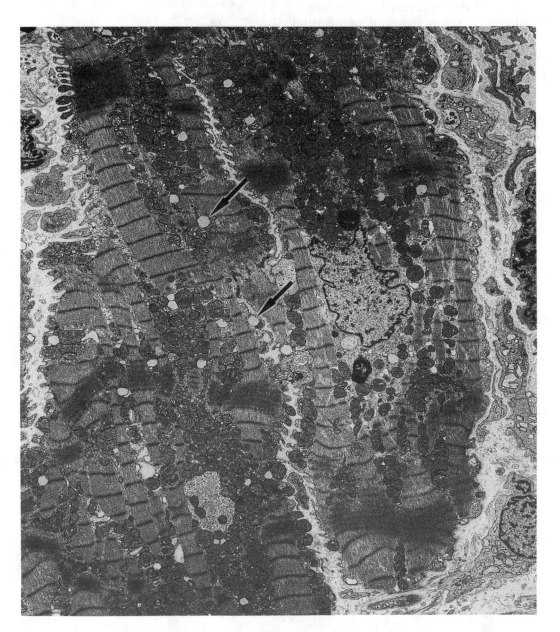

**Fig. 3.**   Electron micrograph of a 15-year-old with lipid droplets in the myocytes (arrows). × 4,570.

ies are undertaken. Once a critical degree of myocardial damage is reached, cardiac function studies may show a rapid change. These studies explain why it is difficult to predict impending heart failure accurately with noninvasive tests, as no change will be detected until clinical heart failure is imminent. Measurements of myocardial function yield a high incidence of nonspecific changes, particularly in the adult population receiving anthracyclines.

In conclusion, anthracycline cardiotoxicity monitored by endomyocardial biopsy is a useful tool for providing a rational basis for dose limitation in adults and children, thereby preventing heart failure. A reliable noninvasive test for monitoring cardiotoxicity, particularly in children, would be preferable, but the endomyocardial biopsy grading system appears to have stood the test of time. It is relatively easy and safe to perform when undertaken by experienced personnel.

## REFERENCES

1. Blum RH, Carter SK: Adriamycin: A new anticancer drug with significant clinical activity. Ann Intern Med 80:249–259, 1974.
2. Lefrak EA, Pittra J, Rosenheim S, Gottlieb JA: A clinicopathologic analysis of Adriamycin cardiotoxicity. Cancer 32:302, 1973.
3. Gottlieb JA, Lefrak EA, O'Bryan RM et al.: Fatal Adriamycin cardiomyopathy. Prevention by dose limitation. Proc Am Assoc Cancer Res ASCO 14:88, 1973.
4. Billingham ME, Mason J, Bristow M, Daniels J: Anthracycline cardiomyopathy monitored by morphological changes. Cancer Treatment Reports 62:865–872, 1978.
5. Bristow M, Mason J, Billingham ME, Daniels J: Doxorubicin cardiomyopathy: Evaluation by phonocardiography, endomyocardial biopsy and cardiac catheterization. Ann Intern Med 88:168–175, 1978.
6. Billingham ME, Bristow M: Evaluation of anthracycline cardiotoxicity: Predictive ability and functional correlation of endomyocardial biopsy. Cancer Treatment Symposia 3:71–76, 1984.
7. Dresdale A, Borror RO, Wesley R, et al.: Prospective evaluation of doxorubicin-induced cardiomyopathy resulting from post-surgical adjuvant treatment of patients with soft tissue sarcomas. Cancer 5:51–60, 1983.
8. Mason JW: Techniques for right and left ventricular endomyocardial biopsy. Am J Cardiol 41:887–892, 1978.
9. Billingham ME, Bristow M, Glatstein E, Mason J, Masek M, Daniels J: Adriamycin cardiotoxicity: Endomyocardial biopsy evidence of enhancement by irradiation. Am J Surg Path 1:17–23, 1977.
10. Billingham ME: Endomyocardial changes in anthracycline-treated patients with and without radiation. In Vaeth J (ed): Front Radiation Therapy Oncology, vol 13. Basel: Karger, 1979, pp 67–81.
11. Rowan R, Masek M, Billingham ME: Ultrastructural morphometric analysis of endomyocardial biopsies: Idiopathic dilated cardiomyopathy, anthracycline cardiotoxicity, and normal myocardium. Am J Cardiovasc Pathol 2:137–144, 1988.
12. Yoshizato T, Edwards WD, Alboliras ET, Hagler DJ, Driscoll DJ: Safety and utility of endomyocardial biopsy in infants, children and adolescents: A review of 66 procedures in 53 patients. J Am Coll Cardiol 15:436–442, 1990.
13. Bristow MR, Mason JE, Billingham ME, Daniels JR: Dose-effect and structure function relationships in doxorubicin cardiomyopathy. Am Heart J 102:709–718, 1981.

# 4. Pathophysiology of Anthracycline Cardiotoxicity

Eugene H. Herman, Ph.D., and Victor J. Ferrans, M.D., Ph.D.

The major side effect that limits anthracycline therapy is severe, cumulative, dose-dependent cardiac toxicity [1]. The first instances of anthracycline-induced cardiotoxicity were recognized during initial clinical trials with daunorubicin [2], but similar alterations were subsequently observed with doxorubicin [1]. This agent induces a spectrum of cardiovascular alterations that includes electrocardiographic changes (nonspecific ST segment and T-wave changes, sinus tachycardia, premature ventricular and atrial contractions, and decreased amplitude of the QRS complex), changes in myocyte morphology, decreased cardiac function, and congestive heart failure [1,3,4]. Pathologic features are similar in humans and experimental animals [3,5,6]. This review discusses the myocardial alterations and the pathogenetic mechanisms of this cardiac toxicity.

## SUBCELLULAR SITES OF ANTHRACYCLINE-INDUCED DAMAGE

Myocyte alterations following exposure to anthracyclines are extremely complex and involve many subcellular organelles, including the sarcolemma, the mitochondria, the nucleus, the nucleolus, the sarcoplasmic reticulum, the lysosomes, and the myofibrils [3,5].

## Sarcolemma

Exposure to doxorubicin results in a variety of functional sarcolemmal abnormalities [7]. However, morphological alterations in structure have been demonstrated in only a few instances [7]. Ultrastructural changes, including aggregation and formation of regular chains of intramembranous particles, have been described in erythrocyte membranes following in vitro exposure to doxorubicin [8]. This finding was interpreted as indicating that molecules of doxorubicin became incorporated into the sarcolemmal lipid bilayer. It has not been determined whether doxorubicin can induce similar changes in the myocyte membrane.

## Mitochondria

Both structural and functional alterations have been reported in myocyte mitochondria of animals given doxorubicin. The most obvious changes following high doses of doxorubicin have been in the mitochondrial structure (swelling, loss of cristae, degeneration and formation of myelin figures) [9]. The induction of overt mitochondrial changes appears to be a function of the manner in which doxorubicin is given, as myocytes in animals dosed chronically have relatively normal-appearing mitochondria [10,11]. In fact, the mitochondrial morphology may be normal in cells showing marked changes in other structures, such as the sarcoplasmic reticulum. In vitro exposure to doxorubicin induces alterations in certain mitochondrial functions, such as their ability to sequester calcium, an effect that could interfere with the control of the intracellular calcium concentration [12]. Doxorubicin reduces the activity of succinoxidase and NADPH oxidase, coenzyme Q10–requiring enzymes [13,14]. Both of these enzymes are important components in the respiratory chain and electron transfer process. The simultaneous administration of coenzyme Q10 was found to partially ameliorate doxorubicin-induced chronic cardiac toxicity in rabbits [15]. Coenzyme Q10, in addition to protecting mitochondrial oxidative function, also stabilizes membranes and is an effective antioxidant. These effects can also contribute to the protection exerted by the agent against doxorubicin cardiotoxicity.

## Nucleus/Nucleolus

Doxorubicin penetrates rapidly into nuclei; by binding to DNA, it interferes with critical nuclear functions and inhibits nucleic acid synthesis [16,17]. Anthracyclines bind to DNA by intercalation, a process by which the drug molecule is inserted into the helical structure of the nucleic acid and thereby interferes with its function. In addition, anthracyclines promote the oxidative destruction of DNA by free-radical mechanisms. The morphologic abnormalities observed in nuclei following administration of doxorubicin are thought to be associated with these actions. Nucleolar segregation takes place in mouse myocardium as early as 10 minutes after a single 10 mg/kg injection of doxorubicin [18]. Nucleolar segregation also occurs in mouse and rat hepatocytes and in rat ventricular myocytes after

large, single doses of doxorubicin [19]. Cardiac myocytes from rats treated with doxorubicin twice a week for 6 weeks had enlarged nuclei and nucleolar organizer regions [20]. The overall significance of these observations is unclear, since nuclear lesions were observed in only a small number of myocytes of patients dying from chronic anthracycline cardiotoxicity [21].

## Sarcoplasmic Reticulum and Myofibrils

The two most prominent characteristics of myocyte degeneration induced by chronic administration of anthracyclines are pale cells and cytoplasmic vacuolization resulting from myofibrillar loss and dilatation of the sarcoplasmic reticulum. Alterations in these organelles develop gradually and may occur in the same cell or in separate cells. Single cells with advanced degenerative changes may be surrounded by intact, normal-appearing cells [3]. The sarcoplasmic reticulum plays a key role in regulating the concentration of intracellular calcium. Doxorubicin causes the release of calcium directly from isolated myocardial sarcoplasmic reticulum [22]. It is likely that alterations in DNA repair, RNA synthesis, and protein replacement are factors in the myofibrillar loss seen in damaged cells following chronic anthracycline administration.

## BIOCHEMICAL EFFECTS OF ANTHRACYCLINES

Anthracyclines may induce biochemical changes capable of producing significant cellular damage. These changes may be due to: (1) conversion of doxorubicin to a toxic metabolite; (2) interaction with cell membranes; (3) release of vasoactive substances; (4) changes in contractile protein; (5) generation of reactive oxygen radicals; and (6) immunological alterations.

## Conversion to Toxic Metabolites

Exposure of isolated cardiac muscle preparations to doxorubicin leads to impaired contractility, relaxation, and compliance [23,24]. The impairment increases with the duration of the exposure [25]. These changes occur simultaneously with the appearance of the C-13 alcohol metabolite doxorubicinol [26]. This metabolite has been found to be more toxic than doxorubicin in isolated cardiac preparations and more active in vitro than doxorubicin in inhibiting the sarcoplasmic reticulum calcium pump [27]. These studies have suggested that the conversion of doxorubicin to doxorubicinol by the cytosolic enzyme anthracycline C-13 ketoreductase might be a factor in the development of chronic anthracycline cardiotoxicity. The anthracycline C-13 ketoreductase enzyme (pH optimum, 8.5) is found in the heart and most other tissues, but not in plasma, and has properties similar to those of a widely distributed group of enzymes, the $NADP^+$ oxidoreductases [27,28]. A second cytosolic anthracycline C-13 ketoreductase, capable of metabolizing doxorubicin, has been identified in human and rat liver [29]. Limited attempts have been made to evaluate the cardiotoxic potential of doxorubicinol in animals. In vivo studies have demonstrated that doxorubicinol, but not doxorubicin, accumulates in myocardial tissue following treatment of rats for a week with multiple injections of doxorubicin [30]. The myocardial alterations observed in this study were attributed to doxorubicinol; however, in studies involving several weeks of dosing, doxorubicinol itself was found to be less cardiotoxic than doxorubicin [31]. In this instance, the difference in cardiotoxic activity might be due to a reduced uptake of the more highly polar doxorubicinol into myocardial cells. Thus, the ultimate role of the C-13 alcohol metabolites, such as doxorubicinol, in anthracycline cardiotoxicity still remains to be determined.

## Interaction With Membranes

Early attempts to characterize a possible doxorubicin–membrane interaction used sonicated liposomes as a model of the phospholipid bilayer [32]. In this system, doxorubicin was noted to alter the fluidity of the liposomal membranes, which contained cardiolipin [32]. This lipid, a component of the mitochondrial inner membrane, is thought to be a key substance in the proper functioning of mitochondrial oxidative activity. Doxorubicin reacts with the negatively charged cardiolipin to form an electrostatic chain complex that can inactivate the electron transport system of mitochondria [33]. Doxorubicin also has been found to inhibit mitochondrial pyruvate transport, an action that may be due to its interaction with cardiolipin in the vicinity of the pyruvate carrier molecule in the mitochondrial membrane [34,35]. This action could also lead to the disruption of myocyte energy production.

Treatment with doxorubicin has produced significant changes in erythrocyte membrane properties, such as the electrical and dielectric charge [36,37]. Thus, interactions with doxorubicin can lead to important alterations in membrane function. These alterations include: (1) increased calcium influx through slow channels [38,39]; (2) altered adenylate cyclase activity [38,39]; (3) inhibition of $Na^+/Ca^{2+}$ exchange or $Ca^{2+}$ ATPase activity [40,41]; and (4) attenuation of $Na^+/K^+$ ATPase activity [41,42]. Interference with sarcolemmal permeability to $Ca^{2+}$ could contribute to the elevation in myocardial calcium concentration found in rabbits treated with doxorubicin [43]. Elevations in intracellular calcium concentrations in other conditions have led to cardiac cellular damage

[44]. However, there is evidence that doxo-rubicin-induced increases in intracellular myocyte calcium could be a result of the cardiotoxicity rather than a cause [45].

## Release of Vasoactive Substances

In acute experiments, monkeys given large doses of daunorubicin, and dogs and rabbits given doxorubicin, had elevated levels of catecholamines and histamine [46,48]. The possibility that anthracycline-induced chronic cardiotoxicity was due to the release of histamine and cat-echolamines was suggested by studies indicating that treatment with pharmacological agents blocking adrenergic (alpha and beta) and histaminergic ($H_1$ and $H_2$) receptors attenuated some of the acute cardiovascular effects [47–50] and reduced myocardial lesions induced by anthracyclines [48,50]. The exact mechanisms responsible for the attenuation of the myocardial lesions are not clear, as the doses of the pharmacologic agents utilized in these studies were considerably in excess of those necessary to block the various receptors. Thus, it is possible that actions other than receptor blockade may have been involved.

Doxorubicin induces the degranulation of, and histamine release from, rat perito-neal mast cells in vitro [51]. Theophylline and disodium cromoglycate, two agents that do not block adrenergic or histaminergic receptors, protect mice against doxorubicin toxicity [52]. These two agents have been reported to prevent the release of histamine from rat peritoneal mast cells. It has been suggested that a decrease in doxorubicin-induced histamine release in vivo is responsible for this protective activity [52]. N-acetylcysteine was also found to interfere with doxorubicin-induced histamine release from rat peritoneal mast cells [52], but this agent has not been effective in ameliorating chronic anthracycline car-

diotoxicity [53,54]. The concept that vaso-active substances are responsible for an-thracycline cardiomyopathy is not consistent with the morphological changes induced by such vasoactive substances in the heart. The cardiac lesions produced by catecholamines [55] and histamine [56] consist of focal necroses that differ considerably from the chronic degenerative lesions produced by the anthracyclines.

## Changes in Contractile Proteins

In addition to myofibrillar lysis, other types of alterations in contractile proteins have been observed in animals given doxorubicin. The interaction with doxorubicin in one study caused G-actin to form unusual filamentous structures, the biophysical properties of which differed from those of the normal actin [57]. The doxorubicin complex with actin also stimulated myosin ATPase activity [57]. Therefore, in vivo binding of doxorubicin to the contractile proteins of myocytes could ultimately alter myocardial contractility.

## Generation of Free Radicals

One of the major pathogenetic mechanisms of anthracycline cardiotoxicity is the generation of toxic free radicals, which could directly damage enzymes, other cellular proteins, and nucleic acids [58]. Free-radical–induced lipid peroxidation can lead to alterations in structural integrity, the transport properties of the membrane, and the activity of membrane enzymes. Myers et al. [58] detected evidence of lipid peroxidation in mouse hearts after administration of doxorubicin. Pretreatment with vitamin E, a free radical scavenger, attenuated the lipid peroxidation and the acute cardiotoxicity induced by doxorubicin [58]. Most mammalian cells have several mechanisms to detoxify oxygen radicals. Cardiac tissue is highly susceptible to the toxic effects of oxygen free radicals because it contains lower concentrations of protective enzymes such as superoxide dismutase, catalase, and selenium-dependent glutathione peroxidase [59,60]. These enzymes function to prevent cellular accumulation of superoxide and hydrogen peroxide. Furthermore, doxorubicin has been found to depress myocardial glutathione peroxidase activity, thereby potentiating its own toxicity [59,60]. At least two mechanisms have been identified by which doxorubicin could initiate the formation of oxygen free radicals.

The first of these mechanisms was initially described by Handa and Sato [61] and involves the formation of a reactive doxorubicin semiquinone radical intermediate by a cytochrome P-450 microsomal enzyme [62]. Subsequently, other oxidoreductases located in the cytoplasm, mitochondria, sarcoplasmic reticulum, and nuclear membrane of myocytes have been found to be capable of converting anthracyclines to a reactive intermediate [60]. The semiquinone intermediate readily donates its unpaired electron to molecular oxygen, forming superoxide, which can lead to the formation of hydrogen peroxide and ultimately the highly reactive hydroxyl radical [62,63].

Since doxorubicin has a high affinity for iron, the formation of a complex between iron and doxorubicin provides a second mechanism to generate reactive oxygen radicals through the conversion of hydrogen peroxide to the hydroxyl radical [64]. This complex has been shown to associate directly with certain cellular components, thus providing the oxygen radicals with almost instantaneous access to target molecules. For example, the doxorubicin–iron complex forms a tertiary complex with DNA that is as reactive as the free drug–metal complex in catalyzing the transfer of an electron from glutathione to oxygen [65]. This tertiary complex is actually much more effective in forming the hydroxyl radical from hydrogen peroxide. The drug–metal complex has been shown to cause oxidative destruction of erythrocyte membranes [66]. It is not clear whether this doxorubicin–iron complex actually has to bind to the membrane in order for this alteration to occur. Myers et al. [64] observed that the membrane damage occurred at very low concentrations of the doxorubicin–iron complex. Free radical scavengers such as N-acetylcysteine and vitamin E are ineffective, both clinically and experimentally, in reducing chronic anthracycline cardiotoxicity. It has been suggested that the drug–metal complex itself can initiate lipid peroxidation without the need for generation of hydroxyl radicals [67]. There is only a very low concentration of free iron in the cytosol for the formation of the drug–metal complex, but doxorubicin has been shown to remove iron from ferritin, its principal intracellular storage pool [68].

Although there is no direct evidence that the drug–metal complex is involved in doxorubicin-induced cardiomyopathy, indirect evidence strongly suggests that iron itself plays a key role in the pathogenesis of the cardiotoxicity. The two most promising cardioprotective agents, ICRF-159 and ICRF-187, both belong to the bisdioxopiperazine family. These compounds are lipophilic derivatives of the metal-complexing agent EDTA and were synthesized as cell membrane–penetrating compounds that upon intracellular hydrolysis would become potential intracellular chelating agents. As indicated below, ICRF-187 attenuates anthracycline toxicity in a variety of animal models. This agent has also been found to be cardioprotective in humans receiving doxorubicin treatment for breast cancer [69,70]. ICRF-187 (the d-isomer) is more water soluble than ICRF-159 (the racemic mixture), and because of this it was utilized in most of the studies.

Initial studies in hamsters showed that ICRF-187 prevented the toxic effects of a single high dose of daunorubicin [71]. ICRF-187 was also protective against anthracyclines, given chronically over a prolonged period. Administration of daunorubicin to rabbits caused myocardial alterations (cytoplasmic vacuolization and loss of myofibrils), which were either absent or reduced in animals pretreated with ICRF-187 [72]. Further studies with ICRF-187 demonstrated effective protection against doxorubicin-induced cardiomyopathy in beagle dogs [73], mice [74], rats [75], guinea pigs [74], and miniature swine [76].

Since the tissues were harvested only 3 weeks after the last dose of doxorubicin in the studies just cited, there was the possibility that cardiomyopathy could have developed more extensively after the termination of the anthracycline therapy, as has been observed in humans [4]. The long-term protective effect of ICRF-187 was evaluated in rabbits given daunorubicin (3.2 mg/kg), alone and in combination with ICRF-187 (25 mg/kg), at 3-week intervals over a 15- or 18-week period (5–6 doses). The severity of the myocardial toxicity was found to be attenuated when the study was terminated at 3 weeks [72] or even 3 months [77] after final treatment. However, in spite of a higher cumulative dose of daunorubicin given to the animals observed at 3 months (19.2 mg/kg) compared to those observed at 3 weeks (16 mg/kg), 71% of the hearts (5 of 7) were free of lesions at 3 months (19.2 mg/kg cumulative daunorubicin dose), as opposed to only 33% (4 of 12) of those observed at 3 weeks (16 mg/kg cumulative daunorubicin dose). Myocardial lesions were apparent in all animals given daunorubicin alone, after 3 weeks or 3 months. It was concluded that ICRF-187 provided true protection, as opposed to causing only a delay in the appearance of the alterations.

Myocardial dysfunction has developed in young adults who underwent success-ful antineoplastic therapy with anthracyclines during childhood without showing immediate cardiotoxicity [78,79]. The mechanism of these long-delayed complications is unknown. It is possible that these late-onset cardiac complications could be prevented by administration of ICRF-187 together with the anthracyclines.

The mechanism by which ICRF-187 attenuates anthracycline-induced cardiotoxic effects has not been completely elucidated. Evidence linking myocyte damage with toxic oxygen free radicals generated by an iron–anthracycline complex has been cited above. ICRF-187 could enter the cell and act as an intracellular iron chelator, thereby interfering with the production of free radicals by the iron–anthracycline complex. A phase I clinical study found evidence of chelating activity, as ICRF-187 caused a 10-fold increase in urinary excretion of iron [80]. Hydrolytic opening of the diketopiperazine rings of ICRF-187 could lead to the formation of a diacid-diamide derivative (ICRF-198), which can remove the iron from the anthracycline complex [81]. The protective activity of ICRF-187 against tissue injury produced by oxygen free radicals has been demonstrated not only with respect to anthracycline-induced cardiomyopathy but also in the pulmonary damage resulting from hyperoxia [82], the pancreatic beta-cell damage induced by alloxan [83], and the pulmonary fibrosis induced by bleomycin [84]. Therefore, these observations could be explained by the concept that the iron chelation produced by the hydrolysis product of ICRF-187 blocks a critical step in the series of reactions leading to the formation of oxygen free radicals that can cause widespread tissue damage.

## Immunological Alterations

Recent investigations have shown that doxorubicin induces many complex alterations in various immune functions, including T-lymphocyte activity [85,86], stimulation of cytolytic T-lymphocyte responses in vitro [87], and increased release of interleukin 2 (IL-2) in rats [88]. Thus, it appears that doxorubicin enhances, rather than suppresses, certain immune functions. It has been suggested that the increase in IL-2 production is related to doxorubicin-induced augmentation of cell-mediated cytotoxicity. Doxorubicin-activated macrophages have been demonstrated to produce interleukin 1 (IL-1), which may induce T-cells to produce IL-2, interferon, or both [89].

Histologic and immunohistochemical studies were made by Zhang et al. [90] to evaluate the quantitative changes in interstitial dendritic cells (antigen-presenting cells), T-helper lymphocytes, T-cytotoxic/suppressor lymphocytes, and macrophages in the hearts of spontaneously hypertensive rats (SHR) treated with doxorubicin, 1 mg/kg per week for 3, 6, 9, or 12 weeks. In addition, an assessment was made of the modifications of the responses of these cell populations when the SHR were given doxorubicin in combination with ICRF-187. The number of interstitial dendritic cells/mm² in sections of the left ventricle was similar in saline-treated control SHR (76 ± 6) and in those treated with ICRF-187 alone (75 ± 2), but was increased markedly (319 ± 33) in animals receiving a total cumulative dose of 12 mg/kg doxorubicin. Pretreatment with ICRF-187 attenuated the doxorubicin-induced increase in numbers of dendritic cells in a dose-dependent manner from 319 ± 33 (doxorubicin alone) to 231 ± 47 at 6.25 mg/kg ICRF-187, 174 ± 11 at 12.5 mg/kg ICRF-187, and 100 ± 16 cells/mm² at 25 mg/kg ICRF-187. Doxorubicin also induced increases in the numbers of T-helper lymphocytes and macrophages, but not of T-cytotoxic/suppressor lymphocytes. These increases were also attenuated by pretreatment with ICRF-187 [90]. These data were interpreted as indicating that doxorubicin cardiotoxicity results in the release of substances that initiate immune reactions involving the antigen-presenting cells of the heart and that such reactions are attenuated by pretreatment with ICRF-187. The relationship of immunological alterations to the development of doxorubicin cardiomyopathy remains to be more fully explored.

# REFERENCES

1. Blum RH, Carter SK: Adriamycin: A new anticancer drug with significant clinical activity. Ann Intern Med 80:249–259, 1974.
2. Tan C, Tasaka T, TU K-P, Murphy L, Karnofsky DA: Daunomycin: An antitumor antibiotic in the treatment of neoplastic disease. Cancer 20:333–353, 1967.
3. Ferrans VJ: Overview of cardiac pathology in relation to anthracycline cardiac toxicity. Cancer Treat Rep 62:955–961, 1978.
4. Von Hoff DD, Layard MW, Basa P, Davis HL Jr, Von Hoff AL, Rozencweig M, Muggia FM: Risk factors for doxorubicin-induced congestive heart failure. Ann Intern Med 31:710–717, 1979.
5. Herman EH: Cardiotoxicity of antineoplastic drugs. In Balazs T (ed): Cardiac Toxicology, vol 2. Boca Raton: CRC Press, 1981, pp 165–186.
6. Powis G: Toxicity of free radical forming anticancer agents. In Powis G, Hacker MP (eds): The Toxicity of Anticancer Drugs. New York: Pergamon Press, 1991, pp 106–151.
7. Tritton TR: Cell surface actions of Adriamycin. Pharmac Ther 49:293–309, 1991.
8. Arancia G, Donelli G: Cell membranes as target for anticancer agents. Pharmacol Res 24:205–217, 1991.
9. Olson HM, Capen CC: Subacute cardiotoxicity of doxorubicin in the rat: Morphologic and ultrastructural investigation. Lab Invest 37:386–394, 1977.
10. Olson HM, Capen CC: Chronic cardiotoxicity of doxorubicin (Adriamycin) in the rat: Morphologic and biochemical investigations. Toxicol Appl Pharmacol 44:605–616, 1978.
11. Jaenke RS: Delayed and progressive myocardial lesions after Adriamycin administration in the rabbit. Cancer Res 36:2558–2966, 1976.
12. Revis N, Marusic N: Effects of doxorubicin and its aglycone metabolite on calcium sequestration by rabbit heart, liver and kidney mitochondria. Life Sci 25:1055–1064, 1979.

13. Iwamoto Y, Hansen IL, Porter TN, Folkers K: Inhibition of coenzyme Q10-enzymes, succinoxidase and NADH oxidase by Adriamycin and other quinones having antitumor activity. Biochem Biophys Res Commun 58:633–638, 1974.

14. Bertazolli C, Sala L, Ballerini L, Wantanabe T, Folkers K: Effect of Adriamycin on the activity of succinate dehydrogenase-coeynzyme Q10 reductase of the rabbit myocardium. Res Commun Chem Pathol Pharmacol 15:797–800, 1976.

15. Bertazolli C, Sala L, Solcia E, Ghione M: Experimental Adriamycin cardiotoxicity prevented by ubiquinone in vivo in rabbits. IRCS Med Sci 3:468, 1975.

16. Arena E, Biondo F, D'Alessandro N, Dusonchet L, Gebbia N, Gerbasi F, Rausa L, Sanguedolce, R: DNA, RNA and protein synthesis in heart, liver and brain of mice treated with daunorubicin or Adriamycin. IRCS Med Sci 2:1053–1061, 1974.

17. Rosenoff SH, Brooks E, Bostick F, Young RC: Alterations in DNA synthesis in cardiac tissues induced by Adriamycin in vivo—relationship to fatal toxicity. Biochem Pharmacol 24:1898–1901, 1975.

18. Lambertenghi-Deliliers G, Zanon PL, Pozzoli EF, Bellini O: Myocardial injury induced by a single dose of Adriamycin: An electron microscopic study. Tumori 62:517–529, 1976.

19. Mirski A, Daskal I, Busch H: Effects of Adriamycin on ultrastructure of nucleoli in the heart and liver cells of the rat. Cancer Res 36:1580–1584, 1976.

20. LeBlanc B, Mompon PR, Esperandieu O, Geffray B, Guillermo C: Nucleolar organizer regions in cardiac lesions induced by doxorubicin. Toxicol Pathol 19:176–183, 1991.

21. Buja LM, Ferrans VJ, Mayer RJ, Roberts WC, Henderson ES: Cardiac ultrastructural changes induced by daunorubicin therapy. Cancer 32:771–788, 1973.

22. Kim DH, Landry III AB, Lee YS, Katz AM: Doxorubicin-induced calcium release from cardiac sarcoplasmic reticulum vesicles. J Mol Cell Cardiol 21:433–436, 1989.

23. Rabkin SW: Interaction of external calcium concentration and verapamil on the effects of doxorubicin (Adriamycin) in the isolated heart preparation. J Cardiovasc Pharmacol 5:848–855, 1983.

24. Hagane K, Akera T, Berlin JR: Doxorubicin: Mechanism of cardiodepressant actions in guinea pigs. J Pharmacol Exp Ther 246:655–661, 1988.

25. Olson RD, Mushlin PS, Brenner DE, Fleischer S, Chang BK, Cusack BJ, Boucek RJ Jr: Doxorubicin cardiotoxicity may be due to its metabolite, doxorubicinol. Proc Natl Acad Sci USA 85:3585–

3589, 1988.

26. Boucek RJ Jr, Olson RD, Brenner DE, Ogunbunmi EM, Inui M, Fleischer S: The major metabolite of doxorubicin is a potent inhibitor of membrane-associated ion pumps. A correlative study of cardiac muscle with isolated membrane fractions. J Biol Chem 262:15851–15856, 1987.

27. Bachur NR, Gee M: Daunorubicin metabolism by rat tissue preparations. J Pharmacol Exp Ther 177;567–572, 1971.

28. Felsted RJ, Richter DR, Bachur NR: Rat liver aldehyde reductase. Biochem Pharmacol 26:1117–1124, 1977.

29. Ahmed NK, Felsted RL, Bachur NR: Daunorubicin reduction mediated by aldehyde and ketone reductases. Xenobiotica 11:131–136, 1981.

30. del Tacca M, Danesi R, Ducci M, Bernardinic, Romanini A: Might adriamycinol contribute to Adriamycin-induced cardiotoxicity? Pharmacol Res Commun 17:1073–1084, 1985.

31. Danesi R, del Tacca M, Bernardinic, Penco S: Exogenous doxorubicinol induces cardiotoxic effects in rats. Eur J Clin Oncol 23:907–913, 1987.

32. Tritton TR, Murphree SA, Sartorelli AC: Adriamycin: A proposal on the specificity of drug action. Biochem Biophys Res Commun 84:802–808, 1978.

33. Fu LX, Waagstein F, Hjalmarson A: A new insight into Adriamycin-induced cardiotoxicity. Int J Cardiol 39:15–20, 1990.

34. Cheneval D, Muller M, Carafoli E: The mitochondrial phosphate carrier reconstituted in liposomes is inhibited by doxorubicin. FEBS Lett 159:123–126, 1983.

35. Paradies G, Ruggierio FM: The effect of doxorubicin on the transport of pyruvate in rat-heart mitochondria. Biochem Biophys Res Commun 156:1302–1307, 1988.

36. Diociaiuti M, Molinari A, Calcabrini A, Arancia G: Electron energy loss spectroscopy analysis of Adriamycin–plasma membrane interaction. J Microsc 164(pt 2):95–106, 1991.

37. Diociaiuti M, Molinari A, Calcabrini A, Arancia G, Bordi F, Cametti C: Alteration of passive electrical properties of Adriamycin-treated red cell membrane deduced from dielectric spectroscopy. Bioelectrochem Bioenerg 26:177–192, 1991.

38. Olson RD, Mushlin PS: Mechanisms of anthracycline cardiotoxicity: Are metabolites involved? In Acosta D (ed): Focus on Molecular, Cellular and In Vitro Toxicology. Boca Raton: CRC Press, 1990, pp 51–81.

39. Singal PK, Panagia V: Direct effects of Adriamycin on the rat heart sarcolemma. Res Common Chem Pathol Pharmacol 43:67–77,

1984.

40. Boucek RJ Jr, Kunkel EM, Graham TP Jr, Brenner DE, Olson RD: Doxorubicinol, the metabolite of doxorubicin, is more cardiotoxic than doxorubicin. Pediatr Res 21:187A, 1987.

41. Tomlinson CW, Godin DV, Rabkin SW: Implications of cellular changes in a canine model with mild impairment of left ventricular function. Biochem Pharmacol 34:4033–4041, 1985.

42. Gosalvez M, Van Rossum GDV, Blanco MF: Inhibition of sodium-potassium-activated adenosine 5'-triphosphate and ion transport by Adriamycin. Cancer Res 39:257–261, 1979.

43. Olson HM, Young DM, Prieur DJ, LeRoy AF, Reagan RL: Electrolyte and morphologic alterations of myocardium in Adriamycin-treated rabbits. Am J Pathol 77:439–545, 1974.

44. Fleckenstein A, Janke J, Doring HS, Pachinger O: Calcium overload as the determinant factor in the production of catecholamine-induced myocardial lesions. In Bajusz E, Rona G (eds): Recent Advances in Studies on Cardiac Structure and Metabolism, vol 2. Baltimore: University Park Press, 1971, pp 455–466.

45. Jensen RA: Doxorubicin cardiotoxicity; contractile changes after long-term treatment in rats. J Pharmacol Exp Ther 2336:197–203, 1986.

46. Herman EH, Vick JA: The acute pharmacological actions of daunomycin in the dog and monkey. Pharmacology 3:291–304, 1970.

47. Herman E, Young R, Krop S: Doxorubicin-induced hypotension in the beagle dog. Agents Actions 8:551–557, 1978.

48. Bristow MR, Sageman SW, Scott RH, Billingham ME, Bowden RE, Kernoff RS, Snidow GH, Daniels TR: Acute and chronic effects of doxorubicin in the dog. The cardiovascular pharmacology of drug-induced histamine release. J Cardiovasc Pharmacol 2:487–515, 1980.

49. Bristow MR, Minobe WA, Billingham ME, Marmor JB, Johnson GA, Ishimoto BM, Sageman WS, Daniels TR: Anthracycline-associated cardiac and renal damage in rabbits: Evidence for mediation by vasoactive substances. Lab Invest 45:157–168, 1981.

50. Bristow MR, Kantrowitz NE, Harrison WD, Minobe WA, Sageman WS, Billingham ME: Mediation of subacute anthracycline cardiotoxicity in rabbits by cardiac histamine release. J Cardiovasc Pharmacol 5:913–919, 1983.

51. Reigel E, Kaliner M, El-Hage A, Ferrans VJ, Kawanami O, Herman EH: Anthracycline-induced histamine release from rat mast cell. Agents Actions 12:431–437, 1982.

52. Klugmann FB, Decorti G, Candussio L, Grill V, Mallardi F, Baldini L: Inhibitors of Adriamycin-induced histamine release in vitro limit Adriamycin cardiotoxicity in vivo. Br J Cancer

54:743–748, 1986.

53. Myers CE, Bonow R, Palmeri S, Jenkins J, Corden B, Locker G, Doroshow J, Epstein S: A randomized controlled trial assessing the prevention of cardiomyopathy by n-acetylcysteine. Sem Oncol 10(suppl 1):53–55, 1983.

54. Herman EH, Ferrans VJ, Myers CE, Van Vleet JF: Comparison of the effectiveness of (±)-1,2-bis(3,5-dioxopiperazinyl-l-yl) propane (ICRF-187) and n-acetylcysteine in preventing chronic doxorubicin cardiotoxicity in beagles. Cancer Res 45:276–281, 1985.

55. Ferrans VJ, Hibbs RG, Walsh JJ, Burch GE: Histochemical and electron microscopic studies on cardiac necrosis produced by sympathomimetic agents. Ann NY Acad Sci 156:309–332, 1969.

56. Franco-Browder S, Guerro M, Gorodezky M, Bravo LM, Aceves S: Lesiones miocardicas producidas por liberadores de histamina en ratas. Arch Inst Cardiol Mexico 30:720–728, 1960.

57. Lewis W, Kleinerman J, Puszkin S: Interaction of Adriamycin in vitro with cardiac myofibrillar proteins. Circ Res 50:547–553, 1982.

58. Myers CE, McGuire WP, Liss RH, Ifrim I, Grotzinger K, Young RC: Adriamycin: The role of lipid peroxidation in cardiac toxicity and tumor response. Science 197:165–167, 1977.

59. Doroshow JH, Locker GY, Myers CE: Enzymatic defenses of the mouse heart against reactive oxygen metabolites. J Clin Invest 65:128–135, 1980.

60. Doroshow JH: Effect of anthracycline antibiotics on oxygen radical formation in rat heart. Cancer Res 43:460–472, 1983.

61. Handa K, Sato S: Simulation of microsomal NADPH oxidation by quinone group containing anticancer chemicals. Gann 67:523–528, 1976.

62. Bachur NR, Gordon SL, Gee MV: A general mechanism for microsomal activation of quinone anticancer agents to free radicals. Cancer Res 38:1745–1750, 1978.

63. Komiyama T, Kikuchi T, Sugiura Y: Generation of hydroxyl radical by anticancer quinone drugs, carbazilquinone, mitomycin C, aclacinomycin A, and Adriamycin, in the presence of NADPH-cytochrome P-450 reductase. Biochem Pharmacol 31:3651–3656, 1982.

64. Myers C, Gianni L, Zweier J, Muindi J, Shina BK, Eliot H: Role of iron in Adriamycin biochemistry. Fed Proc 45:2796–2797, 1986.

65. Eliot H, Gianni L, Myers CE: Oxidative destruction of DNA by the iron–doxorubicin complex. Biochemistry 23:928–936, 1984.

66. Myers CE, Gianni L, Simone CB, Klecker R, Greene R: Oxidative destruction of erythrocyte ghost membrane catalyzed by the doxorubicin–iron complex. Biochemistry 21:1707–1713, 1982.

67. Minotti G, Aust SD: The requirement for iron

(III) in the initiation of lipid peroxidation by iron (II) and hydrogen peroxide. J Biol Chem 262:1098–1104, 1987.

68. Demant EJ: Transfer of ferritin-bound iron to Adriamycin. FEBS Lett 176:97–100, 1984.

69. Speyer JL, Green MD, Kramer E, Rey M, Sanger J, Ward C, Dubin N, Ferrans V, Stecy P, Zeleniuch-Jacquotte A, Wernz J, Feit F, Slater W, Blum R, Muggia F: Protective effect of the bispiperazinedione ICRF-187 against doxorubicin-induced cardiac toxicity in women with advanced breast cancer. N Engl J Med 319:745–752, 1988.

70. Speyer JL, Green MD, Zeleniuch-Jacquotte A, Wernz JC, Rey M, Sanger J, Kramer E, Ferrans V, Hochster H, Meyers M, Blum RH, Feit F, Attubato M, Burrows W, Muggia F: ICRF-187 permits longer treatment with doxorubicin in women with breast cancer. J Clin Oncol 10:117–127, 1992.

71. Herman E, Ardalan B, Bier C, Waravdekar V, Krop S: Reduction of daunorubicin lethality and myocardial cellular alterations by pretreatment with ICRF-187 in Syrian golden hamsters. Cancer Treat Rep 63:89–92, 1979.

72. Herman EH, Ferrans VJ, Jordan W, Ardalan B: Reduction of chronic daunorubicin cardiotoxicity by ICRF-187 in rabbits. Res Commun Chem Pathol Pharmacol 31:85–97, 1981.

73. Herman EH, Ferrans VJ: Reduction of chronic doxorubicin cardiotoxicity in dogs by pretreatment with (+/-)-1,2-bis(3,5-dioxopiperaziny1-1-yl) propane (ICRF-187). Cancer Res 41:3436–3440, 1981.

74. Perkins WE, Schroeder RL, Carrano RA, Imondi AR: Effect of ICRF-187 on doxorubicin-induced myocardial effects in the mouse and guinea pigs. Br J Cancer 46:662–667, 1982.

75. Herman EH, El-Hage A, Ferrans VJ: Protective effect of ICRF-187 on doxorubicin-induced cardiac and renal toxicity in spontaneously hypertensive (SHR) and normotensive (WKY) rats. Toxicol Appl Pharmacol 92:42–53, 1988.

76. Herman EH, Ferrans VJ: Influence of Vitamin E and ICRF-187 on chronic doxorubicin cardiotoxicity in miniature swine. Lab Invest 49:69–77, 1983.

77. Herman EH, Ferrans VJ: Pretreatment with ICRF-187 provides long-lasting protection against chronic daunorubicin cardiotoxicity in rabbits. Cancer Chemother Pharmacol 16:102–106, 1986.

78. Lipshultz SE, Colan SD, Gelber RD, Perez-Atayde AR, Sallan SE, Sanders SP: Late cardiac effects of doxorubicin therapy for acute lymphoblastic leukemia in childhood. N Engl J Med 324:808–815, 1991.

79. Steinherz LJ, Steinherz PG, Tan TCT, Heller G, Murphy L: Cardiac toxicity 4 to 20 years after completing anthracycline therapy. J Am Med Assoc 266:1672–1677, 1991.

80. Von Hoff DD, Howser D, Lewis BJ, Holcenberg J, Weiss RB, Young RC: Phase I study of ICRF-187 using a daily for 3 days schedule. Cancer Treat Rep 65:249–252, 1981.

81. Hasinoff BB: The interaction of the cardio-protectant agent ICRF-187(+)-1,2-bis(3,5-dioxopiperazinyl-l-yl)propane): Its hydrolysis product (ICRF-198) and other chelating agents with the Fe (III) and Ca (II) complexes of Adriamycin. Agents Actions 26:378–385, 1989.

82. Herman EH, Zhang J, Zhang TM, Ferrans VJ: Attenuation of bleomycin-induced pulmonary and renal toxicity in mice by ICRF-187. FASEB J 4(3):A615,1990.

83. El-Hage A, Herman EH, Yang GC, Crouch RC, Ferrans VJ: Mechanisms of the protective activity of ICRF-187 against alloxan-induced diabetes in mice. Res Commun Chem Pathol Pharmacol 52:341–360, 1986.

84. Fukuda Y, Herman EH, Ferrans VJ: Effect of ICRF-187 on the pulmonary damage induced by hyperoxia in the rat. Toxicology 74:185–202, 1992.

85. Ehrke MJ, Ryoyma K, Cohen SA: Cellular basis for Adriamycin-induced augmentation of cell-mediated cytotoxicity in culture. Cancer Res 44:2497–2504, 1984.

86. Maccubin DL, Whitman JA, Taniguchi N, Mace KF, Ehrke MJ, Mihich E: Comparison of Adriamycin induced imminomodulation with that of the noncardiotoxic anthracycline 5-iminodaunorubicin. Int J Immunopharmacol 10:317–323, 1988.

87. Huber SA: Doxorubicin-induced alterations in cultured myocardial cells stimulate cytolytic T-lymphocyte responses. Am J Pathol 137:449–456, 1990.

88. Abdul Hamied TA, Turk JL: Enhancement of interleukin-2 release in rats by treatment with bleomycin and Adriamycin in vivo. Cancer Immunol Immunother 25:245–249, 1987.

89. Hart DNJ, Fabre JW: Demonstration and characterization of 1a-positive dendritic cells in the interstitial connective tissue of rat heart and other tissues, but not brain. J Exp Med 153:347–361, 1981.

90. Zhang J, Herman EH, Ferrans VJ: Dendritic cells in the hearts of spontaneously hypertensive rats treated with doxorubicin with or without ICRF-187. Am J Pathol (in press).

# 5. Radiation-Related Heart Disease: Risks After Treatment of Hodgkin's Disease During Childhood and Adolescence

Steven L. Hancock, M.D., and Sarah S. Donaldson, M.D.

A broad spectrum of cardiac diseases has been identified as possible sequelae of high-dose irradiation of the mediastinum [1]. Pericardial diseases, including acute pericarditis during mediastinal irradiation, delayed acute pericarditis and pericardial effusions, constrictive pericarditis, and pancarditis (pericardial and myocardial fibrosis), were the first identified and most frequently documented of the radiation-induced or radiation-associated heart diseases [2–10]. Early changes in the techniques of radiation therapy were thought to have decreased the severity of this problem [11,12]. Electrocardiographic abnormalities and conduction defects have also been occasionally reported [2,13–18]. There has been controversy about the contribution of mediastinal irradiation to valvular heart disease [1,6,13,19,20] and to premature coronary artery disease [13,14,21–25] after mediastinal irradiation. Recent studies, however, support increased risks for death from acute myocardial infarction in adult populations [26–28]. The risk for significant cardiac disease has generally been considered low following irradiation during childhood and adolescence [28,29], but recent analyses of patients treated for Hodgkin's disease at Stanford University indicate a high incidence of cardiac abnor-malities among patients treated with full-dose irradiation before 21 years of age. They have high relative risks for deaths from heart diseases—especially acute myocardial infarction. This chapter reviews those findings and the background information regarding radiation-associated cardiac diseases.

## PATIENT POPULATION

Stanford University provided initial therapy for 2,232 patients with Hodgkin's disease between January 1961 and April 1991. Six hundred and thirty-five of these (351 males, 284 females) were under 21 years of age at the initiation of treatment and were analyzed for subsequent cardiac diseases. Their ages ranged from 2 to 20 years (average: 15.4 years); follow-up averaged 10.3 years. Initial treatment consisted of radiation alone in 311 patients, 78 of whom required chemotherapy for recurrent Hodgkin's disease (mecloreth-amine, vincristine, and procarbazine [MOP] in 56 patients; doxorubicin, bleomycin, vinblastine, and dacarbazine [ABVD] either alone or alternating with MOP in six patients, and other regimens in 16 patients). Three hundred and six patients received initial combined irradiation and chemotherapy, with MOP(P) in 162 patients (prednisone was included in cycles 1 and 4 if the patient had not received mediastinal irradiation), PAVe (procarbazine, melphalan, and vinblastine) in 57, ABVD alone or alternating with MOP(P) or PAVe in 66, or other regimens in 22 patients. Eighteen patients received initial chemotherapy alone, but 12 of them received subsequent mediastinal irradiation during treatment of recurrent disease.

The extent of irradiation varied: 244 patients received total lymphoid irradiation; 208 received subtotal lymphoid irradiation that omitted the pelvic lymph nodes; 165 received limited-field irradiation, 51 of whom received no mediastinal irradiation [30]. Radiation doses tended to increase with increasing age at treatment, while chemotherapy use decreased with increasing age. The nine patients treated before 5 years of age received chemotherapy and mediastinal radiation doses that did not exceed 30 Gy. Of the 56 patients treated from 5 through 9 years of age, 77% received chemotherapy, and 39% had mediastinal irradiation doses that exceeded 30 Gy. Sixty-nine percent of the 146 patients treated from 10 through 14 years of age received chemotherapy, and 48% were given more than 30 Gy to the mediastinum. Sixty percent of the 423 patients who were 15 through 21 years of age received chemotherapy, and 91% had more than 30 Gy to the mediastinum. Seventy-one percent of the patients under 21 years of age were given 40 Gy or more to the mediastinum.

All of the patients received megavoltage irradiation on a 4.8 or 6 MV linear accelerator. Treatment before 1971 included most of the cardiac silhouette, and fraction size varied from 2.2 to 2.75 Gy per day, with anterior and posterior fields treated on alternate days. After 1970, most mediastinal fields included subcarinal blocking that limited the radiation dose to much of the ventricular myocardium to 30 Gy. Since the mid-1970s, both anterior and posterior fields were treated daily, with fraction sizes limited to 1.5 to 1.8 Gy per day, and most patients under 17 years of age were treated on combined modality protocols that limited the radiation fields and doses to 15 to 25 Gy [31].

Patients were followed for both recurrence of Hodgkin's disease and potential treatment complications and for intercurrent diseases at intervals that increased from bimonthly during the first posttreatment year to annually after 5 years. Follow-up information was sought from the patients, their parents, and referring and follow-up physicians by letter and health questionnaire when 2 years elapsed since the last contact. Follow-up of the 635 patients represents 6,564 person-years of observation. Cardiac abnormalities and deaths were collected from computerized complication records that were entered after each follow-up visit and by review of individual patient records and correspondence. Records of heart disease care were requested from outside institutions, when necessary. Risks were assessed by Kaplan-Meier plots [32], with the Gehan test [33] used to assess significance in comparisons, and by relative risks: the ratio of the observed to the expected number of cases. The expected number of cardiac deaths was calculated by compiling person-years of observation for each patient from the date of initial treatment for Hodgkin's disease to the last follow-up date or date of death and then applying age-, sex- and race-specific annualized mortality rates obtained from United States Decennial Life Tables [34] using the methods of Monson and exact Poisson probabilities to obtain tests of significance and confidence intervals for the relative risks [35]. Relative risk values with confidence intervals that included a relative risk of 1.0 or less were not considered significantly elevated. Absolute risk, the excess number of cases expected in a population of defined size, was calculated by subtracting the expected number of events from the observed number of events, dividing by the accumulated person-years of observation, and multiplying by $10^4$ to give rates per 10,000 person-years of observation. Patients who relapsed after initial radiation alone or chemotherapy alone contributed person-years after relapse to the combined treatment group in analyses of risk according to treatment. There were 12 deaths from cardiac diseases and 103 nonfatal cardiac abnormalities recorded.

## RISK OF HEART DISEASE DEATHS

The overall risk of death from cardiac diseases after Hodgkin's disease has not been well established in existing reports. The 12 heart disease deaths identified in the 635 children and adolescents represented an 8.8% actuarial risk of death from heart disease after 22 years from treatment and a relative risk of 29.6 (95% confidence interval [CI]: 16.0 to 49.3). The absolute risk was 17.7 excess cases per 10,000 person-years. The risk for heart disease death did not vary significantly by gender. The actuarial risk of cardiac death tended to be higher in males than females (M: 13.8%; F: 4.3%, $P = 0.9$). However, the relative risk (RR) of a heart disease death tended to be higher in females than males (F: four events; RR: 36.3; 95% CI: 11.4 to 87.8; M: eight events; RR: 27.2; 95% CI: 12.6 to 51.7). The risk for cardiac death was similar for those treated with radiation alone or with radiation and adjuvant or subsequent chemotherapy. The actuarial risk of cardiac death was 10.2% for radiation alone and 12% with combined therapy after 22 years

from treatment ($P = 0.3$). The relative risk was 28.1 with radiation alone (95% CI: 12.3 to 55.5) and 37.1 with combined therapy (95% CI: 13.6 to 82.5). The risk of a cardiac death was not elevated among the small number of patients who received chemotherapy alone or radiation that excluded the mediastinum.

## RISKS OF ACUTE MYOCARDIAL INFARCTION

Seven of the 12 deaths were due to acute myocardial infarction. The Kaplan-Meier risk of death from this cause was 6% after 22 years from treatment and the relative risk was 41.5 (95% CI: 18.1 to 82.1). Neither gender nor the addition of chemotherapy to irradiation significantly altered the risk for myocardial infarction death, the relative risk for which tended to be higher among females than males (F: RR: 70.4; 95% CI: 11.7 to 233; M: RR: 35.6; 95% CI: 13 to 79). It was higher among those treated with radiation alone than with chemotherapy and radiation (radiation alone: RR: 52.2; 95% CI: 21 to 109; radiation and chemotherapy: RR: 21.1; 95% CI: 0 to 104). The Kaplan-Meier risk was not significantly greater for radiation alone than chemotherapy and radiation (radiation alone: 8.8%; radiation and chemotherapy: 0.4%; $P = 0.59$). The relative risks for myocardial infarction death were significantly elevated for those patients 5 to 9 years out from therapy and remained similarly elevated throughout more than 20 years after irradiation. There was no suggestion of a prolonged latent period between treatment and increased risk for myocardial infarction death.

Three additional patients have survived acute myocardial infarctions in this population. One of these underwent cardiac transplantation for ischemic cardiomyopathy; another required resection of a left ventricular aneurysm and revascularization of the left anterior descending coronary artery. The Kaplan-Meier risk of a fatal or nonfatal acute myocardial infarction in this population reached 8.2% after 22 years. Three other patients have undergone coronary artery revascularization an average of 21 years after mediastinal irradiation.

The relative risk of acute myocardial infarction death in this population of patients treated as children and adolescents is substantially higher than previously reported risks after treatment of Hodgkin's disease. An earlier analysis from Stanford [26] evaluated 326 patients who were 18 years of age or older (average: 29 years of age) and were entered into randomized comparisons of radiation alone or radiation and meclorethamine, vincristine, procarbazine, and prednisone chemotherapy. The relative risk of death from acute myocardial infarction was 3.2 (95% CI: 1.5 to 5.8). Boivin et al. [28] recently reported a case-cohort study of 4,665 Hodgkin's disease patients treated at several institutions between 1940 and 1985 and followed an average of 7 years. The age-adjusted relative risk of acute myocardial infarction death was 2.56 (95% CI: 1.11 to 5.93) following mediastinal irradiation and 0.97 (95% CI: 0.53–1.77) after chemotherapy. The age distribution was not specified in that study, but the authors reported a higher risk for mediastinal irradiation at age 60 or more (RR: 2.16) than at age 40 or less (RR: 1.84) or from age 40 through 59 (RR: 1.23). The higher risks observed in the younger Stanford population suggest greater susceptibility to premature coronary artery disease in younger patients exposed to mediastinal radiation doses above 40 Gy (particularly those patients between 15 and 21 years of age). However, the higher risks may reflect greater uncertainty in the population statistics that estimate the expected risk of acute myocardial infarction or other heart disease deaths in a young, general population where such events are probably rare. The United States Decennial Life Tables for 1979 to 1981 were used to estimate expected rates in the normal population. Because the risk of acute myocardial infarction death has declined since 1981, these should represent conservative (i.e., high) estimates of the expected risks, supporting the premise of greater susceptibility to coronary injury with younger age [36]. None of the studies assessing the risk of acute myocardial infarction death has shown an enhancing effect of chemotherapy on the acute myocardial infarction risk associated with mediastinal irradiation. In the population under 21 years of age, such analysis is confounded by potential differences in the extent of cardiac irradiation (since chemotherapy prior to irradiation may decrease the volume of irradiated myocardium), by the lower mediastinal irradiation doses that many patients under 17 years of age received, and by the evolving, increasingly conservative radiation techniques used in more recently treated patients. The 10 patients who had lethal or nonlethal acute myocardial infarctions received radiation doses of 42 to 45 Gy; seven were treated without subcarinal blocking. The events in the three other patients suggest that either lower dose irradiation confers risk or that limited subcarinal blocking alone may not adequately protect the proximal coronary arteries. Although the latency analyses in this population suggest equivalent risk of myocardial infarction death from 5 to more than 20 years after irradiation, those patients who were treated with more conservative mediastinal fields and radiation doses, with or without chemotherapy, may demonstrate an elevated risk with further follow-up.

## RISKS FROM OTHER CARDIAC DISEASE

Five of the patients treated before 21 years of age have died of cardiac diseases other than acute myocardial infarction. Two deaths were attributed to radiation pericarditis or pancarditis at 2.6 and 19 years after irradiation, one resulted from valvular endocarditis at 12 years, one from valvular surgery at 20 years, and one from deterioration of congenital heart disease 4.5 years after irradiation. The relative risk of death from heart diseases other than myocardial infarction was 21.2 (95% CI: 7.8 to 47.2). The risk did not vary by gender (M: RR: 19.5; 95% CI: 4.9 to 53.2; F: RR: 24.5; 95% CI: 4.1 to 81). However, the risk tended to be higher for those treated with radiation and chemotherapy than with radiation alone (radiation alone: RR: 7.4; 95% CI: 0.0 to 36.5; radiation and chemotherapy: RR: 45.8; 95% CI: 14.4 to 111; Kaplan-Meier risks after 20 years: radiation alone: 1.6%; radiation and chemotherapy: 12.5%; $P = 0.1$). There were no trends in the latency of risk for death from heart diseases other than myocardial infarction, with events and risk similarly distributed from less than 5 to 20 years after irradiation.

In addition to the two deaths attributed to radiation pericarditis or pancarditis, there were a variety of other pericardial diseases in the Stanford population treated before 21 years of age. Twelve patients underwent pericardiectomy for symptomatic constrictive pericarditis an average of 7.4 years after Hodgkin's disease therapy (range: 10 months to 16.8 years). The actuarial risk of requiring pericardiectomy reached 4% at 17 years of follow-up.

Forty patients had diagnoses of acute pericarditis based upon typical positional chest pain, friction rubs on auscultation, and/or cardiomegaly or effusions on chest radiographs or cardiac ultrasound examinations. Eight of these arose during the course of mediastinal irradiation. None required interruption of treatment, and none of the patients have had subsequent pericardial or cardiac disease.

Thirty patients developed these pericarditis syndromes from 4 months to 18 years after irradiation (average: 6 years); two developed acute pericarditis after abrupt withdrawal of an incidental course of corticosteroid medications 7 and 15 years after irradiation. Three patients have a diagnosis of cardiomyopathy, two of whom had poor residual cardiac function despite pericardiectomy or valvular surgery.

As previously reported, significant pericardial disease is most common after treatment of large volumes of the heart to high doses [1–10]. Greenwood et al. [7] reported a 7% incidence of severe constrictive pericarditis among 86 children irradiated to the mediastinum and associated the problem with high-dose, orthovoltage radiation. All of the patients treated as children or adolescents at Stanford who required pericardiectomy or died of pericarditis or pancarditis had high-dose mediastinal irradiation with little or no cardiac blocking. Ten were irradiated prior to the introduction of subcarinal blocking. Two received chemotherapy and radiation to large volumes of the heart for extensive mediastinal involvement by Hodgkin's disease.

The "delayed" acute pericarditis syndromes of positional chest pain, fever, and friction rubs and effusions or asymptomatic pericardial effusions noted on follow-up have also been associated with high radiation doses to the heart. Carmel and Kaplan [12] reported a 20% incidence of these syndromes after irradiation of the whole pericardium to 40 Gy or more and noted a decline in incidence to 7.5% with partial cardiac shielding and 2.5% with subcarinal blocking after 30 to 35 Gy. Twenty of the 30 children and adolescents who developed these pericarditis syndromes after irradiation were treated prior to the introduction of subcarinal blocking in 1971. Most of these episodes were self-limited, although five patients underwent pericardiectomy from 3 months to 5 years after the episode of "acute pericarditis" or 2 to 17 years after mediastinal irradiation. The "recall" of radiation pneumonitis and pericarditis observed in two patients after abrupt discontinuation of corticosteroids has also been previously described [37], although the two cases observed in the younger population demonstrate a very prolonged period of susceptibility. The patient who had "recall pericarditis" after corticosteroid withdrawal nearly 15 years after mediastinal irradiation had a previous, spontaneous episode of acute pericarditis 7 years earlier.

## VALVULAR HEART DISEASE

Two of the cardiac deaths among those irradiated as children and adolescents were attributed to valvular heart disease. The impact of irradiation on a third patient's death from congenital heart disease was uncertain. Two others required aortic valve replacement and a third required mitral valve replacement 15 to 21 years after irradiation. Morton et al. [6] reported two early cases of aortic regurgitation in patients with radiation pericarditis and Brosius et al. [13] noted thickened valvular endocardium in 12 of 16 autopsies of patients irradiated to high doses before 27 years of age, but the contribution of radiation to the development of valvular heart disease remains uncertain [1,19,20]. Twenty-nine of the patients irradiated before 21 years of age at Stanford have developed apparently new heart murmurs, on average 14 years after medi-

astinal irradiation. Some of these may represent flow murmurs attributable to impaired chest-wall development from high-dose irradiation at an early age. The extent to which these murmurs represent significant valvular pathology and the contribution of irradiation to accelerated valvular disease remains uncertain.

## CONDUCTION ABNORMALITIES

Three of the patients irradiated before the age of 21 have developed conduction abnormalities on electrocardiogram from 14.5 to 24 years after irradiation. These included left or right bundle branch block and a bradyarrhythmia with a high-grade atrioventricular block that required pacemaker implantation at age 32. One patient reported a diagnosis of paroxysmal atrial tachycardia with episodic tachyarrhythmias 1.5 years after irradiation. Conduction abnormalities are well documented, occasional late sequelae of high-dose mediastinal irradiation [2,13–18]. Their incidence varies widely in studies that have systematically screened small populations of patients for cardiac abnormalities after mediastinal irradiation and correlates with the dose and volume of cardiac irradiation. None were found by Green et al. [29] in 28 patients irradiated between 5 and 17 years of age and evaluated 19 to 182 months after mediastinal doses of 2,034 to 3,978 cGy by anterior and posterior fields. Similarly, Morgan et al. [38] found normal electrocardiograms in 25 Hodgkin's disease patients who were evaluated 5 to 16 years after 40 Gy to a mantle field with subcarinal block placement at 30 Gy. Seven patients had abnormal resting electrocardiograms among 48 patients who underwent cardiopulmonary screening at Stanford from 1 to 15 years after mantle treatment of 42.8 to 55 Gy during the era of routine subcarinal blocking [39]. The abnormalities included one complete and four incomplete right bundle branch blocks and two first-degree atrioventricular blocks. The highest incidence of electrocardiographic abnormalities (as well as pericardial and myocardial injury) has been reported after mantle treatments that were administered solely from the anterior field. Gottdiener et al. [40] found electrocardiographic abnormalities in 12 of 25 patients who were screened, on average, 10.9 years after anterior field irradiation. In a study by Pohjola-Sintonen et al. [14], 46% of 28 patients had abnormal electrocardiograms when screened more than 5 years after anteriorly treated mantles. Four of those patients had a right bundle branch block and four had first-degree atrioventricular block.

## SUMMARY

Radiation-induced heart disease remains a significant problem for Hodgkin's disease patients treated with 40 Gy or more to the mediastinum using alternating AP/PA fields with heart blocks and appears to be a particularly high risk in patients treated before 21 years of age. The relative risk of a cardiac death in this population at Stanford was 29.6, and the relative risk of death from acute myocardial infarction was 41.5. These risks became significantly elevated soon after irradiation (within 5 to 10 years for acute myocardial infarction death and within 5 years for other cardiac death) and remained elevated throughout more than 20 years of follow-up. The actuarial risk of a fatal or nonfatal acute myocardial infarction has reached 8.2% after 22 years of follow-up.

In addition to the high risks for death from premature coronary artery disease and other cardiac diseases, there has been substantial late morbidity in patients who received high-dose irradiation at an early age. The actuarial risk of requiring pericardiectomy for constrictive pericarditis has reached 4% after 18 years of observation. The risk for radiation-induced valvular heart disease is difficult to assess. Two patients irradiated before 21 years of age died of valvular heart disease at long intervals after irradiation, and several others have required valvular surgery. A substantial number of cardiac or flow murmurs have been described in the late follow-up period in these patients, although their significance is unclear. These and several electrocardiographic changes have been recorded in the routine, general follow-up care of young patients treated for Hodgkin's disease and probably represent an underestimate of changes that remain subclinical, thus far. Systematic screening with electrocardiography, echocardiography, exercise testing (with or without radionuclides), and angiography, if indicated, would likely identify additional potential problems. The benefits to an asymptomatic individual from such screening, the optimal interval to an initial screen or frequency of screenings, and the possible risks from invasive intervention because of abnormalities found in screening have not been defined. These issues have kept such investigations controversial [41]. The high relative risks for cardiac disease deaths and the large number of clinical abnormalities that have followed high-dose mediastinal irradiation indicate the need for sensitive consideration of potential cardiac symptoms and signs among treated patients and for prompt evaluation and care, when required. The findings also support the current studies that seek to limit the extent and dose of irradiation in children and adolescents. During the last decade, children with Hodgkin's disease typically received combined modality therapy with lower radiation doses (15 to 25 Gy) to more limited volumes with treatment of both opposed fields each day. These improved techniques are expected to decrease many of the risks associated with previous Hodgkin's disease treatment approaches. However, the late effects of such treatment strategies will take many more years to evaluate.

## ACKNOWLEDGMENTS

The authors thank Mrs. Anna Varghese for data management and analysis and Ms. Marge Keskin for assistance in preparing the manuscript. This work was supported in part by NIH grant CA 34233.

## REFERENCES

1. Stewart JR, Fajardo LF: Radiation-induced heart disease: An update. Prog Cardiovasc Dis 27:173–194, 1984.
2. Rubin E, Camara J, Grayzel DM, Zak FG: Radiation-induced cardiac fibrosis. Am J Med 34:71–75, 1963.
3. Cohn KE, Stewart JR, Fajardo LF, Hancock EW: Heart disease following radiation. Medicine 46:281–298, 1967.
4. Stewart JR, Cohn KE, Fajardo LF, Hancock EW, Kaplan HS: Radiation-induced heart disease. Radiology 89:302–310, 1967.
5. Stewart R, Fajardo LF: Dose response in human and experimental radiation-induced heart disease: Application of the nominal standard dose (NSD) concept. Radiology 99:403–408, 1971.
6. Morton DL, Glancy DL, Joseph WL, Adkins PC: Management of patients with radiation-induced pericarditis with effusion: A note on the development of aortic regurgitation in two of them. Chest 64:291–297, 1973.
7. Greenwood RD, Rosenthal A, Cassady R, Jaffe N, Nadas AS: Constrictive pericarditis in childhood due to mediastinal irradiation. Circulation 50:1033–1039, 1974.
8. Applefeld MM, Wiernik PH: Cardiac disease after radiation therapy for Hodgkin's disease: Analysis of 48 patients. Am J Cardiol 51:1679–1681, 1983.
9. Mill WB, Baglan RJ, Kurichety P, Prasad S, Lee JY, Moller R: Symptomatic radiation-induced pericarditis in Hodgkin's disease. Int J Radiat Oncol Biol Phys 10:2061–2065, 1984.
10. Cameron J, Oesterle SN, Baldwin JC, Hancock EW: The etiologic spectrum of constrictive pericarditis. Am Heart J 113:354–360, 1987.
11. Kaplan HS: Hodgkin's disease. Cambridge: Harvard University Press, , 1972, pp 279–296.
12. Carmel RJ, Kaplan HS: Mantle irradiation in Hodgkin's disease: An analysis of technique, tumor eradication, and complications. Cancer 37:2813–2825, 1976.
13. Brosius FC, Waller BF, Roberts WC: Radiation heart disease. Analysis of 16 young (aged 15 to 33 years) necropsy patients who received over 3,500 rads to the heart. Am J Med 70:519–530, 1981.
14. Pohjola-Sintonen S, Totterman KJ, Salmo M, Siltanes P: Late cardiac effects of mediastinal radiotherapy in patients with Hodgkin's disease. Cancer 60:31–37, 1987.
15. Cohen SI, Bharati S, Glass J, Lev M: Radiotherapy as a cause of complete atrioventricular block in Hodgkin's disease. Arch Intern Med 141:676–679, 1981.
16. Totterman KJ, Pesonen E, Siltanen P: Radiation-related chronic heart disease. Chest 83:875–878, 1983.
17. Borrel E, Wolf JE, Page E, et al.: Une complication rare de la radiotherapie thoracique: Le bloc auriculoventriculaire. A propos d'une observation et revue de la litterature. Ann Cardiol Angeiol 39:351–355, 1990.
18. Slama MS, Le Guludec D, Sebag C, et al.: Complete atrioventricular block following mediastinal irradiation: A report of six cases. PACE 14:1112–1118, 1991.
19. Fajardo LF, Stewart JR, Cohn KE: Morphology of radiation-induced heart disease. Arch Pathol 86:512–519, 1968.
20. Fajardo LF, Stewart JR: Pathogenesis of radiation-induced myocardial fibrosis. Lab Invest 29:244–257, 1973.
21. Boivin JF, Hutchison GB: Coronary heart disease mortality after irradiation for Hodgkin's disease. Cancer 49:2470–2475, 1982.
22. Donaldson SS, Kaplan HS: Complications of treatment of Hodgkin's disease in children. Cancer Treat Rep 66:977–989, 1982.
23. Annest LS, Anderson RP, Li W, Hafermann MD: Coronary artery disease following mediastinal radiation therapy. J Thorac Cardiovasc Surg 85:257–263, 1983.
24. Strender LE, Lindahl J, Larsson LE: Incidence of heart disease and functional significance of changes in the electrocardiogram 10 years after radiotherapy for breast cancer. Cancer 57:929–934, 1986.
25. Lederman GS, Sheldon TA, Chaffey JT, Herman

TS, Gelman RS, Coleman CN: Cardiac disease after mediastinal irradiation for seminoma. Cancer 60:772–776, 1987.

26. Hancock SL, Hoppe RT, Horning SJ, Rosenberg SA: Intercurrent death after Hodgkin disease therapy in radiotherapy and adjuvant MOPP trials. Ann Intern Med 109:183–189, 1988.

Corrections in: Hancock SL, Cox RS, Rosenberg SA: Deaths after treatment of Hodgkin disease. Ann Intern Med 114:810, 1991.

27. Cosset JM, Henry-Amar M, Pellae-Cosset B, et al.: Pericarditis and myocardial infarctions after Hodgkin's disease therapy. Int J Radiat Oncol Biol Phys 21:447–449, 1991.

28. Boivin JF, Hutchison GB, Lubin JH, Mauch P: Coronary artery disease mortality in patients treated for Hodgkin's disease. Cancer 69:1241–1247, 1992.

29. Green DM, Gingell RL, Pearce J, Panahon AM, Ghoorah J: The effect of mediastinal irradiation on cardiac function of patients treated during childhood and adolescence for Hodgkin's disease. J Clin Oncol 5:239–245, 1987.

30. Kaplan HS: Hodgkin's Disease, 2nd ed. Cambridge: Harvard University Press, 1980, pp 366–407.

31. Donaldson SS: Hodgkin's disease in children. Semin Oncol 17:736–748, 1990.

32. Kaplan EL, Meier P: Nonparametric estimation from incomplete observations. Am Stat Assoc 53:457–481, 1958.

33. Gehan EA: A generalized Wilcoxon test for comparing arbitrarily singly-censored samples. Biometrika 52:203–223, 1965.

34. National Center for Health Statistics: U.S. Decennial Life Tables 1979 through 1981. Vol 2(5):12–15, 1985.

35. Monson RR: Analysis of relative survival and proportional mortality. Comput Biomed Res 7:325–332, 1974.

36. Manson JE, Tosteson H, Ridker PM, et al.: The primary prevention of myocardial infarction. N Engl J Med 326:1406–1416, 1992.

37. Castellino RA, Glatstein E, Turbow WM, et al.: Latent radiation injury of lungs or heart activated by steroid withdrawal. Ann Intern Med 80:593–599, 1974.

38. Morgan GW, Freeman AP, McLean RG, et al.: Late cardiac, thyroid, and pulmonary sequelae of mantle radiotherapy for Hodgkin's disease. Int J Radiat Oncol Biol Phys 11:1925–1931, 1985.

39. Watchie J, Coleman CN, Raffin TA, et al.: Minimal long-term cardiopulmonary dysfunction following treatment for Hodgkin's disease. Int J Radiat Oncol Biol Phys 13:517–524, 1987.

40. Gottdiener JS, Katin MJ, Borer JS, Bacharach SL, Green MV: Late cardiac effects of therapeutic mediastinal irradiation: Assessment by echocardiography and radionuclide angiography. Med Intelligence 308:569–572, 1983.

41. Hancock EW: Heart disease after radiation. N Engl J Med 308:588, 1983.

# 6. The Use of Echocardiography and Holter Monitoring in the Assessment of Anthracycline-Treated Patients

Steven E. Lipshultz, M.D., and Steven D. Colan, M.D.

The limitation of cumulative anthracycline dosage over the past 15 years has resulted in a low incidence (<1%) of congestive heart failure during chemotherapy [1]. However, the late cardiac implications of such therapy are only beginning to be understood [2–10]. Sensitive cardiac testing of survivors of childhood cancer treated with anthracyclines reveals an alarming incidence of progressive abnormalities at a point of relatively early follow-up (6 years) in children who otherwise would look forward to decades of active, productive life [4]. Late congestive heart failure, high-grade symptomatic arrhythmias, and sudden death have been noted both in patients who did and in those who did not have congestive heart failure during therapy [2–10].

Because of the effectiveness of current therapy for childhood cancer, the population of survivors is continuously expanding. By the year 2000, about 1 out of every 900 young adults in the United States will be a survivor of malignant disease in childhood or adolescence [11]. There are an estimated 77,300 survivors of childhood cancer diagnosed in the first 15 years of life using 1992 figures [11–14]. If 40% received anthracycline therapy, then nearly 31,000 survivors of childhood cancer may be at risk for late cardiotoxicity; if newly diagnosed cases up to the age of 21 years are included, the total number of anthracycline-treated survivors in the United States is greater than 43,500 [13].

We review these cardiac problems in more detail because there is not a clear appreciation of the late cardiac complications that may be encountered by this first generation of successfully treated survivors, and because this is a growing population. The extent to which the cure of a potentially fatal childhood malignancy results in another serious or even fatal disease remains to be determined. Our goal is to minimize late cardiotoxicity by (1) preventing cardiac damage during chemotherapy in children and (2) altering the course of progressive cardiotoxicity in previously treated survivors.

## ASSESSMENT OF VENTRICULAR FUNCTION: DEFINITIONS AND LIMITATIONS

### Fractional Shortening Versus Contractility

It is important to understand how the health of cardiac muscle is assessed. Left ventricular contractility is one important measurement. Fractional shortening and ejection fraction, evaluated at rest by either echocardiographic or nuclear medicine techniques, are commonly used indi-

*Cardiac Toxicity After Treatment for Childhood Cancer*, pages 45–62, ©1993 Wiley-Liss, Inc.

ces to assess ventricular systolic performance. The latter is governed by the intrinsic ability of the myocardium (contractility), the loading conditions under which the myocardium is working, and, to a lesser extent, the heart rate [15–18]. However, cardiac performance reflects all the determinants of ventricular function, not just contractility, and these commonly used indices do not differentiate contractility changes from alterations in loading conditions [15–25]. When the heart rate, left ventricular preload, and left ventricular afterload are all normal, the trends observed by using these load-dependent indices may approximate those observed for left ventricular contractility. However, in populations in which the loading conditions are known to be abnormal, such as in children treated for cancer [2–4], standard indices of function cannot be relied on to indicate the contractile state of the myocardium. In such populations, the loading conditions must be measured for a true assessment of the contractile state.

The limitations of load-dependent measurements are inherent in the indices and are independent of the measurement technique used. There is no reason to expect that an ejection fraction properly measured by radionuclide angiography is better or worse, more or less sensitive, or more or less specific than fractional shortening properly measured from an echocardiogram. Each of these is a measure of fiber shortening, which is inherently dependent on preload, afterload, and contractility.

Recognition of the limitations of these load-dependent indices in this population has led to an increased use of more invasive and expensive means of assessing these same indices under exercise or pharmacologic myocardial stress. These tests are used in an effort to unmask cardiac dysfunction that was occult at rest [5,6,8,26]. Dynamic stress studies detect a larger number of patients with abnormal load-dependent contractility than do routine studies. They nonetheless remain incapable of discriminating between the effects of ventricular loading conditions and the effects of ventricular contractility. In fact, they may even introduce other variables likely to impair exercise during therapy, including neuropathy and pulmonary toxicity.

As a result of these limitations, we have employed an index of left ventricular contractility that is independent of preload and incorporates afterload. It is also noninvasive and relatively easy to perform. This index, called the stress–velocity index, is the relationship between the rate-corrected velocity of circumferential fiber shortening and end-systolic wall stress [21,27]. The stress–velocity index incorporates measurements of contractility, afterload, and preload, enabling their independent contributions to abnormalities of ventricular performance to be assessed. We have used this index for 9 years now and have found it useful for cardiac monitoring both during therapy for childhood cancer and during late serial evaluations of cardiovascular status, as well as for monitoring the effects of cardiac interventions [3,4,28–32].

Left ventricular fractional shortening and contractility are not equivalent. Treatment decisions may differ according to which measurement was used to assess the health of the left ventricle. This report does not explore the implications of these differences for clinical management, but only establishes that there are differences and that clinicians should be aware of the limitations of the measurements they may be using. However, there are data that demonstrate why contractility is a better measure of cardiac health than fractional shortening. Borow et al. [33] evaluated left ventricular contractility indices in adults with dilated cardiomyopathy. The stress–velocity index was the most physiologically appropriate for assessing pharmacologically induced changes in ionotropic state that were accompanied by complex alterations in loading conditions. In patients with aortic regurgitation requiring surgery, contractility and loading conditions provide a better prediction of postoperative ventricular function than load-dependent indices alone [34–38]. A patient with aortic regurgitation and depressed fractional shortening will more likely return to a normal fractional shortening after valve replacement, if the cause was afterload excess, than will a patient with depressed contractility. In children with renal failure, depressed fractional shortening is common [39]. However, this reduced fractional shortening is almost exclusively due to extrinsic factors, and such patients may be misclassified as having cardiomyopathy, particularly before preload reduction with dialysis.

Loading-condition abnormalities may be either extrinsic or intrinsic, and understanding the difference may affect therapeutic options. Afterload is affected by extrinsic factors such as blood pressure, arterial compliance, and ventricular outflow obstruction, and by intrinsic factors such as inadequate hypertrophy, excess hypertrophy, and ventricular dilation (Fig. 1) [40]. Preload is affected by extrinsic factors such as altered myocardial relaxation and compliance (Fig. 2) [40]. Indeed, an altered ionotropic state itself, through secondary effects on left ventricular geometry and chamber pressure, may influence preload and afterload (Fig. 3) [40].

Characterizing a patient as having cardiomyopathy implies that something is intrinsically wrong with the myocardium. Fractional shortening does not discriminate between intrinsic and extrinsic effects on ventricular function and is therefore of limited use in determining which patients have cardiomyopathy [41]. The ability to diagnose cardiomyopathy cor-

rectly is particularly important, as symptomatic idiopathic cardiomyopathy carries high mortality: 63% 1-year and 34% 5-year survival rates in one study of children [42]. In a more recent study of children >2 years of age with dilated cardiomyopathy, the 2-year survival rate was 20%, and all 12 patients were dead within 9 years after presentation, regardless of whether congestive heart failure was present at the time of diagnosis [43]. Studies of congestive cardiomyopathy among adults report 15% to 60% annual mortality rates, with 60% to 75% dead within 5 years after presentation [44,45].

Somatic growth is associated with alterations in myocardial mechanics. In normal children, afterload rises markedly with age and body size (Fig. 4), most dramatically during the first few years, and contractility falls [27]. Fractional shortening also changes during childhood, owing to the age-related increase in afterload and decrease in contractility (Fig. 5) [27]. For example, the normal fractional shortening for neonates ranges from 35% to 45% (±2 SD), whereas by 20 years of age, the range is 28% to 38%. This age-related change in fractional shortening implies that using a single non-age-adjusted fractional shortening criterion for adjusting chemotherapy is almost certainly inappropriate.

### Mildly Depressed Ventricular Function

Limitations of load-dependent indices are particularly significant in survivors of childhood cancer. When an arbitrary fractional shortening close to normal is used to define depressed function (e.g., 28%), fractional shortening and contractility correlate poorly [4]. In one study, we found that the exclusive use of fractional shortening less than 28% resulted in 43% of children with depressed fractional shortening being misclassified owing to a very

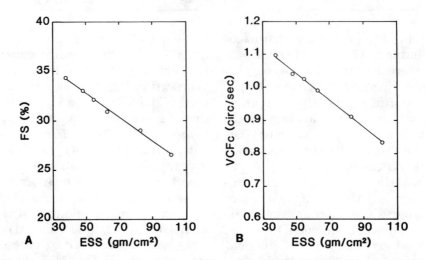

**Fig. 1.** Relation of end-systolic wall stress (ESS) to **(A)** left ventricular percent fractional shortening (FS) and to **(B)** rate-corrected velocity of fiber shortening (VCFc). A graded increase in afterload (ESS) was induced by an infusion of methoxamine in a single individual. Methoxamine increased the blood pressure slowly. The dramatic effect of increasing afterload resulting in a decrease in systolic function can be seen clearly. Details of the data collection method are given in references 21 and 40.

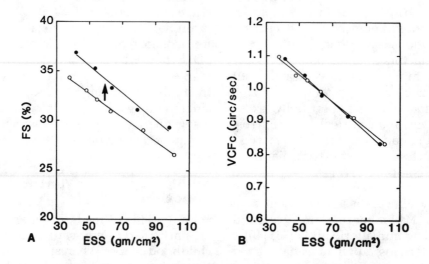

**Fig. 2.** Relation of end-systolic wall stress (ESS) to **(A)** left ventricular percent fractional shortening (FS) and to **(B)** rate-corrected velocity of fiber shortening (VCFc) before (open circles) and after (closed circles) dextran infusion in an individual over a wide range of afterload conditions achieved by methoxamine infusion. Arrow indicates shift following dextran infusion. Preload augmentation with dextran resulted in a significant upward shift of the stress-shortening relation in a manner similar to that seen with positive inotropic intervention at any level of afterload, indicating that changes to fractional shortening at different afterload states result from changes in preload. However, there was no significant change in the stress–velocity index before and after dextran infusion, indicating that it is an index of contractility that is independent of preload. Details of the data-collection method are given in references 21 and 40.

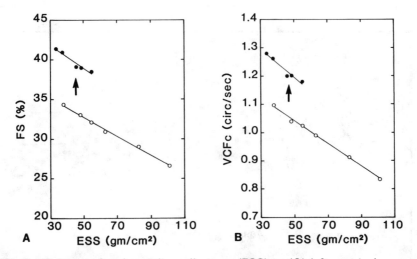

**Fig. 3.** Relation of end-systolic wall stress (ESS) to (**A**) left ventricular percent fractional shortening (FS) and to (**B**) rate-corrected velocity of fiber shortening (VCFc) before (open circles) and after (closed circles) dobutamine infusion in an individual over a wide range of afterload conditions achieved by methoxamine infusion. Arrows indicate shifts following dobutamine infusion. Both indices respond to changes in contractility. Details of the data-collection method are given in references 21 and 40.

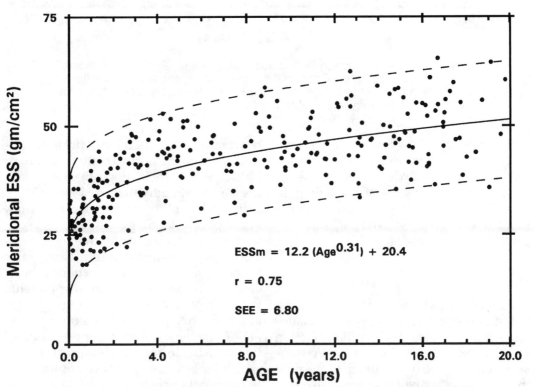

$$ESSm = 12.2\,(Age^{0.31}) + 20.4$$

$$r = 0.75$$

$$SEE = 6.80$$

**Fig. 4.** Age-related rise in meridional end-systolic wall stress (ESS). The relation of ESS (afterload) to age was best predicted by a power function. The nonlinear curve fit (solid line) and 95% confidence intervals (dotted lines) are shown, and the equation, correlation coefficient (r), and standard error of the estimate (SEE) are given for each. Details of the data-collection method are given in reference 27.

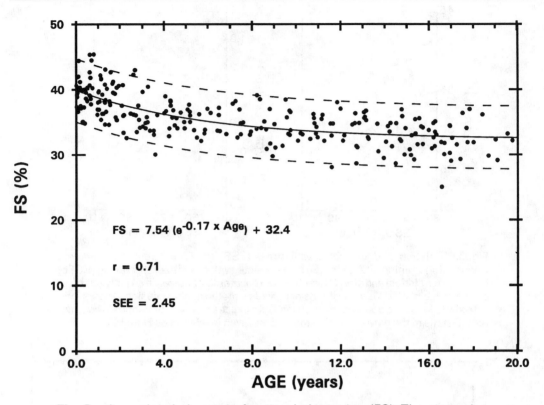

$$FS = 7.54 (e^{-0.17 \times Age}) + 32.4$$

$$r = 0.71$$

$$SEE = 2.45$$

**Fig. 5.** Age-related change in fractional shortening (FS). The regression line, confidence intervals, exponential decay equation, correlation coefficient (r), and standard error of the estimate (SEE) are shown. Details of the data-collection method are given in reference 27.

high incidence of abnormal loading conditions [46,47]. It is also not correct to say that all patients with depressed contractility have reduced fractional shortening. In fact, 25% of patients with normal or enhanced fractional shortening had depressed contractility [46,47].

## Congestive Heart Failure

Discrepancies between fractional shortening and contractility appear to matter less when a patient's ventricular function is at an extreme. Although either measurement may be useful much of the time in that setting, we have demonstrated that 25% of human immunodeficiency virus (HIV)-infected children with congestive heart failure did not have depressed contractility. Having normal contractility may influence how their congestive heart failure is subsequently managed [46,47].

In addition to ventricular function, knowledge of loading conditions and contractile state enables better treatment decisions to be made. Although ventricular function, as assessed by fractional shortening, was depressed in all our patients with congestive heart failure, the causes and thus the appropriate therapy varied [46,47]. In some patients, depressed function was due to abnormal contractility, for which ionotropic agents are appropriate. In other patients, depressed function was due to excessive afterload, for which afterload-reducing agents, such as angiotensin-converting enzyme inhibitors, are indicated. A more rational selection of appropriate cardiac therapeutic agents in symptomatic patients is needed, since many of these agents have been associated with significant adverse reactions [48,49].

## Ventricular Function During Chemotherapy

Load-dependent indices of ventricular function at rest have not proved reliable in detecting depressed left ventricular contractility or in predicting children likely to develop congestive heart failure during treatment for cancer [50,51]. It is not necessarily true that once fractional shortening is abnormal, the patient has sustained clinically significant myocardial damage. A variety of factors completely unrelated to the health of the heart muscle cell can cause fractional shortening to be abnormal, which is precisely why methods must be used that can discriminate between muscle cell damage and other factors. Factors contributing to differences between load-dependent ventricular function and contractility during chemotherapy include anemia, fever, volume infusions, central nervous system disease (including seizures), autonomic imbalance, renal failure, and malnutrition. For example, fever causes tachycardia and cutaneous vasodilation, resulting in reduced systemic resistance and afterload. Even a mildly abnormal ventricle might exhibit a normal ejection fraction under these conditions. Conversely, renal failure, by causing high blood pressure and increased intravascular volume, raises both afterload and preload. Even a normal ventricle in this case may have a low ejection fraction, not because of myocardial toxicity but because of excessive load on the ventricle. The influence of loading conditions thus may lower the sensitivity and specificity of the

ejection-phase indices for detecting abnormal ventricular function due to anthracycline. Moreover, the absence of hypertension, fever, or anemia, for example, does not necessarily make fractional shortening a reliable measure of contractility, either. For example, healthy long-distance runners, who would be expected to have a normal left ventricular fractional shortening at rest, have a significantly reduced fractional shortening due to reduced preload at rest, even though their contractility is normal [52]. This finding would not have been obvious without an assessment of contractility and loading conditions.

## Ventricular Function in Long-Term Survivors of Childhood Cancer

Similar to cardiac function during chemotherapy, changes in fractional shortening or ejection fraction in long-term survivors who have been treated with doxorubicin do not predict late congestive heart failure. In one study, we found that 41% of doxorubicin-treated long-term survivors of childhood leukemia with depressed fractional shortening had normal or enhanced ventricular contractility [4]. Abnormal loading conditions contributed to the fractional shortening and contractility measurements not being equivalent. More than 50% of the total study population had elevated afterload, owing largely to progressive thinning of the left ventricular wall with increasing age and growth. Therefore, load-dependent indices of ventricular function do not portray accurately the status of ventricular contractility in late survivors as well.

In summary, the high incidence of abnormal loading conditions in children treated for cancer precludes the use of load-dependent ejection-phase indices, particularly fractional shortening, to assess contractile state. Measurements of load-independent contractility and specific loading conditions allow a more accurate determination of clinical status and may lead to better clinical management of children treated for cancer.

## SCREENING

Recommendations have been made to monitor children for cardiotoxicity at intervals during the course of anthracycline chemotherapy for cancer and for late cardiotoxicity by means of a detailed cardiac testing protocol [53]. These recommendations generally encompass echocardiographic evaluation, radionuclide investigations of cardiac function, endomyocardial biopsy, electrocardiography, and Holter monitoring. Protocols such as these proceed on the assumption that if cardiac monitoring reveals an abnormal finding, chemotherapy should be withheld even from patients who are otherwise asymptomatic from a cardiac perspective, in the hope that clinically significant heart disease can be avoided or reduced. We believe that these recommendations should be carefully considered for two reasons: (1) Potentially life-saving chemotherapy may be inappropriately withheld and (2) a costly intensive cardiac monitoring program may be undertaken in the absence of scientific justification. Although many aspects of these programs are controversial, a single, fundamental issue represents both the central message and the problem it represents. The recommendations contend that by following the proposed methods of cardiac assessment and discontinuing anthracycline therapy in patients who manifest a fall in left ventricular function, it is possible to reduce the incidence of cardiotoxicity without adversely affecting cancer cure rates. Thus, the two primary hypotheses are that cancer cure rates will not decrease and that cardio-

toxicity will be less common or severe.

At present, no evidence exists to support the concept that any of the recommendations for cardiac monitoring and subsequent dose modification result in a net benefit to patients. In fact, it is entirely possible that such a program could result in lower overall survival, with an increase in cancer-related deaths exceeding the reduction in cardiac deaths. The examples in Figure 6 illustrate possible differences in the balance between death from disease recurrence and death from cardiotoxicity with different doses of anthracyclines.

## Assessment of Cardiac Rhythm, Function, and Structure During Pediatric Anthracycline Treatment for Cancer as a Predictor of Subsequent Clinical Congestive Heart Failure

**Electrocardiography.** Work in the 1970s demonstrated that electrocardiography has no prognostic value in determining which patients will go on to clinical congestive heart failure [1,50,51,54–57]. Some reports have suggested that $QT_c$ prolongation is a sign of cardiac involvement [58,59], but no study has demonstrated that the presence of a prolonged $QT_c$ interval results in subsequent clinical congestive heart failure. Ventricular late potentials, noted by electrocardiography, are thought to represent delayed depolarization of the myocardium and are observed after myocardial infarction and in patients with cardiomyopathy. A signal-averaged electrocardiogram has been used to study the occurrence of ventricular late potentials in children during or after chemotherapy. This has not been found to correlate with anthracycline therapy or dosage or with the presence of diminished fractional shortening [60]. The authors con-

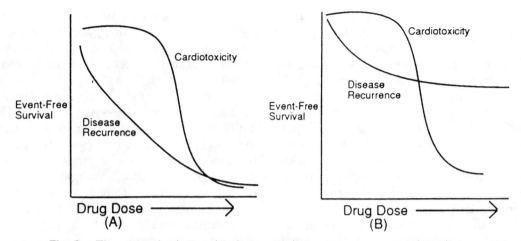

**Fig. 6**.   Theoretical relationship between disease recurrence and cardiotoxicity. In panel **A**, for a substantial gain in recurrence-free survival, the risk of cardiomyopathy is significantly increased. Panel **B** illustrates a very different scenario. The risk of disease recurrence is relatively constant over the area that encompasses little risk of cardiotoxicity to that with substantial risk. Hence, there would be little gain in recurrence-free survival but a substantially increased risk of cardiotoxicity as a function of drug dose. It is likely that the slopes of these curves will differ by cancer diagnosis, since recurrence-free survival is diagnosis-dependent; moreover, the incidence rates of different types of cancer peak at different ages, an important factor in calculating the risk of cardiotoxicity. (Used with permission of Jeffrey P. Krischer, Ph.D.)

cluded that late ventricular potentials were not helpful for the early detection of myocardial injury in this population. Preliminary work suggests that in long-term survivors of childhood cancer treated with anthracyclines, the presence of ventricular tachycardia relates to the subsequent onset of late congestive heart failure [30]. However, no detailed analysis of ventricular tachycardia as a predictive factor has been made in long-term survivors, and no data in patients receiving therapy relate the presence of arrhythmias to subsequent congestive heart failure.

**Echocardiography.**   Measures of ventricular function that are dependent on loading conditions, such as fractional shortening or ejection fraction, have shown no predictive value for identifying patients who subsequently develop congestive heart failure following anthracycline therapy. Our work suggests that a low

fractional shortening within 1 year of completion of anthracycline correlates with sustained depressed ventricular contractility as determined by echocardiography 6 years after completing therapy, but no patient in that study developed late congestive heart failure who did not have it initially [4]. In addition, elsewhere we have reported other patients who developed late congestive heart failure as an initial event [3]. Steinherz et al. [7] similarly suggested that late depressed fractional shortening correlates with early depressed fractional shortening at the completion of therapy. The problem with load-dependent measures of ventricular performance is that depressed function only occasionally correlates with true cardiac muscle damage and depressed contractility. The use of load-independent indices of left ventricular contractility such as the stress–velocity index may improve this predictive capacity, but such indices have been employed in only a preliminary fashion [61]. It is not yet known whether they can predict which patients may subsequently develop congestive heart failure.

**Radionuclide studies.** Resting radionuclide studies of ejection fraction suffer from the same problems as load-dependent indices assessed by echocardiography. They are influenced by a variety of noncardiac factors and do not provide an accurate evaluation of left ventricular contractility when such measures as afterload, preload, and heart rate are abnormal. Radionuclide tests discriminate poorly between different types of dilated cardiomyopathy [62].

Results from exercise radionuclide studies are even more difficult to interpret. When endomyocardial biopsy and right heart catheterization results were compared with exercise radionuclide ejection fraction, McKillop et al. [63] found that the addition of exercise improved the sensitivity of the test from 53% to 89%. This was gained at the expense of a significant decrease in specificity, from 75% to 41%, however [63]. In addition, the disadvantages of exercise ventriculograms include the fact that many patients cannot undertake it owing to age (children <7 years) or to an inability to exercise to an adequate level (e.g., acute illness or amputation). During chemotherapy, children have difficulty attaining normal exercise performance. The effects of ongoing therapy, including such factors as malnutrition, fever, or anemia (which certainly adversely affects load-dependent left ventricular performance at rest and with exercise), tend to affect exercise testing adversely. Vincristine neuropathy, bleomycin pulmonary toxicity, central nervous system insults (including seizures, strokes, and autonomic dysfunction), or limb-salvage procedures are other conditions that would affect exercise testing at that stage. Some

of these factors may have a lasting effect on exercise performance, and these factors would have to be considered before exercise abnormalities could be attributed to anthracyclines.

Moreover, more than 30% of normal children have abnormal exercise radionuclide studies, so abnormal studies may be meaningless. Parrish et al. [64] evaluated continuous staged supine exercise on a bicycle ergometer using multigated radionuclide ventriculography at rest and during each exercise stage in normal children. They found that 10 of 31 (32%) normal children had a resting left ventricular ejection fraction of ≤55% and 10 (32%) had a change in the left ventricular ejection fraction with exercise of ≤5%. These results differ from adult studies and suggest that a significant percentage of normal children would be abnormal both at rest and during exercise if this technique and usual adult standards were used. These techniques and standards are probably even more inappropriate for children treated for cancer [65].

**Endomyocardial biopsy.** Billingham and Bristow [66] and others have recommended endomyocardial biopsy as a means of assessing acute toxicity in adults undergoing anthracycline chemotherapy. However, there appears to be a variable relationship between the histologic abnormalities and the functional consequences, with at least some investigators reporting a weak predictive capacity for the clinical significance of the myocardial biopsy. Isner et al. [67] demonstrated in a controlled study that a high percentage of patients with abnormal endomyocardial biopsies had no congestive heart failure; furthermore, a high percentage of patients with normal endomyocardial biopsies had clinical congestive heart failure. Their results suggest that this procedure may be of no value for routine monitoring of anthracycline cardiotoxicity in adults. In addition to the usual risks associated with endo-myocardial biopsy, the disadvantages of serial biopsy are of particular importance in the pediatric population and certainly limit the utility of this tool. We are not aware of any study of endomyocardial biopsy in children as a predictor for subsequent clinical congestive heart failure.

## Selective Dose Reduction of Anthracyclines, Cardiotoxicity, and Survival

In summary, at present it has not been adequately documented that any of these tests are good predictors of myocardial injury after anthracycline therapy. Clearly, further investigations into this issue are warranted. It is certainly possible that other indices or methods may provide a suitable measure of the magnitude of cardiotoxicity. Even then, though, further issues must be considered, as discussed below. There are no data at this point to indicate that reducing the anthracycline dosage selectively in response to abnormal cardiac studies during the course of therapy lessens either the incidence of subsequent clinical congestive heart failure or early mortality from heart disease in excess of that which can be attained by arbitrary dosage limits in all subjects. More important, we do not know how such a modification of therapy in asymptomatic patients affects the percentage of patients who go into complete remission or remain in remission. Patients, for example, may experience transient abnormal cardiac studies during therapy. Following recommendations similar to those cited above [53] would have resulted in termination of therapy prematurely for approximately 30% of patients [50,51]. What is not known is whether this reduction will result in a decrease in the incidence of congestive heart failure developing around the time of therapy, which is already very low (<1%)

for most pediatric protocols. In at least one study [50,51] testing a cardiac monitoring program such as that described here, none of the 22% to 31% of patients who would have had their doxorubicin stopped early under these recommendations had an adverse cardiac outcome.

Next, if a reduction in congestive heart failure during therapy should be demonstrated, we do not know how that will balance against the possibility that more patients may die from not going into complete remission secondary to a reduced cumulative anthracycline dosage. No data exist at this point comparing the balance between these two very important factors. Theoretically, if it were possible to reduce the dosage of anthracycline without reducing the cure rates, then why not simply reduce the dosage for everyone? Implicit in the entire discussion is the assumption that higher dosages result in higher cancer cure rates; otherwise, one could and should reduce the total dosage, independent of any change in cardiac function. Therefore, it must be assumed that a program of cardiac monitoring that will reduce the total dosage will result in lower cure rates. In fact, the only reasonable approach to this problem is to accept the concept that we are dealing with a balance between adverse cancer outcomes and adverse cardiac outcome: Reducing one will increase the other.

## Congestive Heart Failure During Therapy and in Long-Term Survivors

Our work has suggested that some patients develop late congestive heart failure as a result of chronically elevated afterload related to abnormally thin ventricular walls, presumed secondary to myocyte loss during anthracycline therapy [4]. This mechanism does not appear to be related to the mechanism responsible for the congestive heart failure that develops during therapy. In contrast to the histologic changes observed with acute toxicity, our patients with afterload excess and subsequent late congestive heart failure have histologically healthy-looking cardiac myocytes with significant hypertrophy and minimal fibrosis. Therefore, employing current regimens as a package to prevent both early and late congestive heart failure may be overly simplistic and ineffective.

## Summary of Data on Cardiac Monitoring

Our current state of knowledge would suggest that recommendations are premature for modifying anthracycline dosages in response to prospective monitoring of cardiac function during anthracycline therapy for childhood cancer in patients without clinical evidence of cardiotoxicity. We strongly agree that cardiac monitoring to reduce the incidence of clinical congestive heart failure is a laudable goal, but such recommendations must be based on data that examine both sides of the equation. Moreover, there are no data to support any cardiac methodology as a valid predictor of clinical congestive heart failure in this population, nor is there any data regarding the effect of early termination of therapy on the efficacy of cancer therapy.

## Costs and Benefits

The financial cost of cardiac monitoring would be quite high, and the potential increased cost of fewer cured patients cannot be assessed at this time. In 1992, the average prices at our institution are in excess of $1,000 for a nuclear medicine scan or an echocardiographic evaluation of ventricular function, $500 for a Holter monitor study, and $5,000 for an endo-

myocardial biopsy. According to the published recommendation, a patient receiving doxorubicin at 30 mg/m$^2$ to a cumulative dosage of 360 mg/m$^2$ would receive 10 echocardiograms, two radionuclide scans, and two electrocardiograms if every study were completely normal during therapy and during the first year of follow-up after completing anthracycline therapy [53]. This series amounts to more than $15,000 per patient. If these recommendations were followed on all newly diagnosed patients 21 years of age or under treated with anthracyclines, the national cost for routine cardiac monitoring alone would exceed $48 million a year.

On the benefit side of the equation, a reduction in both early and late clinically significant cardiotoxicity is the desired goal, but it is not now known what might be done to reduce the incidence. The most important change in therapy to avoid early cardiotoxicity has been to reduce the cumulative anthracycline dosage. This has, indeed, reduced the incidence of congestive heart failure during therapy. A review of the first 1,800 patients treated with doxorubicin shows that 30% to 40% of the patients who received a total dosage of 600 to 1,000 mg/m$^2$ developed congestive heart failure. This is to be compared with 1% of patients whose total dosage was ≤500 mg/m$^2$ [1]. In the recent paper by Steinherz et al., recommending serial cardiac monitoring and concomitant dosage modification, the authors described a 0.4% incidence of congestive heart failure during therapy [53]. Studies at our institution have shown that changes in fractional shortening or ejection fraction do not predict which patients will develop congestive heart failure during chemotherapy [50,51], so that we do not modify the anthracycline dosage without clinical evidence of congestive heart failure as well. In fact, most patients have not had serial routine measurements during chemotherapy unless they are on research protocols that specifically measure ventricular function. With that as an institutional policy, our incidence of acute congestive heart failure over the past 10 years has remained similar to that of other centers, regardless of whether they have practiced dosage modification. For example, over the past 10 years, 878 children have been treated with doxorubicin for acute lymphoblastic leukemia (ALL) on Dana Farber Cancer Institute protocols (81-01, 85-01, and 87-01). Only one patient (0.1%) developed congestive heart failure during therapy or in the first year after therapy [68,69]. Steinherz et al. [7] noted that monitoring and dose modification did not appear to have a major impact on late follow-up measurements of fractional shortening when compared to our unmonitored population; 23% of their patients had abnormal fractional shortening compared with 28% of ours. In addition, the disease-free survival rate in our children treated for ALL is comparable to the highest reported anywhere. For newly diagnosed patients treated with anthracyclines throughout the United States, incidence figures of less than 1% would suggest that 12 to 20 patients a year would develop congestive heart failure during therapy. It is uncertain that spending over $48 million a year for extensive cardiac monitoring will significantly reduce this number.

But the large unknown is the effect of monitoring and subsequent dosage modification on overall survival and late cardiotoxicity. The effects of monitoring and dosage adjustment on overall survival rates are not known, and the implementation of these recommendations will only impede our ability to address this issue. Only controlled trials can address the issue of how disease-free survival rates are affected by cardiac monitoring and dosage modification. Comparisons of pooled survival rates are not valid, because most centers modify dosage in the recommended manner and oncologic patient management is not the same at different institutions. Thus, the measurable and nonmeasurable costs of monitoring and dosage modification appear high, and the benefit not at all clear. This kind of monitoring, however, might be of value in a well-designed research study to assess its value for predicting early and late congestive heart failure and its effect on overall survival.

## RESULTS OF STUDIES OF CARDIAC FUNCTION IN LONG-TERM SURVIVORS OF CHILDHOOD CANCER

We recently reported [4] that doxorubicin therapy in childhood impairs myocardial growth in a dosage-related fashion and results in a progressive increase in left ventricular afterload, sometimes accompanied by reduced contractility. Fifty-seven percent of 115 children who had been treated for ALL with doxorubicin 1 to 15 years earlier, and in whom the disease was in continuous remission, had abnormalities of left ventricular afterload or contractility. The cumulative dosage of doxorubicin was the most significant predictor of abnormal cardiac function. Sixty-five percent of patients who received 228 to 550 mg/m$^2$ (median, 360 mg/m$^2$) had increased afterload (59% of patients), decreased contractility (23%), or both. Increased afterload was due to reduced ventricular wall thickness, not to hypertension or ventricular dilatation. In multivariate analyses, the only significant predictive factors were a higher cumulative dosage, which predicted depressed contractility, and an age of less than 4 years at treatment, which predicted increased afterload. Afterload increased progressively in 24 of 34 patients (71%) evaluated serially. Reported symptoms correlated poorly with indices of exercise tolerance or ventricular function. Eleven patients had congestive heart failure within 1 year of treatment; five of them had recurrent heart failure 3.7 to 10.3 years after completing treatment. No patient had late heart failure as a new event, although we have seen this with other patients [3]. We hypothesize that the loss of myocytes during doxorubicin therapy in childhood may result in inadequate left ventricular mass and clinically important heart disease in later years. Other models of chronically elevated afterload demonstrate secondary depression of left ventricular contractility [70].

Depressed contractility is noted in many long-term survivors of childhood ALL treated with doxorubicin and may contribute to adverse late cardiac outcomes. Depressed contractility relates to high cumulative doxorubicin dosages; yet even at lower cumulative dosages, late cardiotoxicity is also a problem. Because other predictors are not known, we examined the effects of gender and dose rate on late depressed contractility and found it present in 23% of the patients, some of whom had congestive heart failure [32]. Although girls represented 50% of the study sample and had a cumulative doxorubicin dosage (361 mg/m$^2$) similar to the overall group, all eight patients with late isolated depressed contractility were girls. In fact, 70% (16/23) of patients with depressed contractility and either normal or increased afterload were girls. Doxorubicin doses of 30 mg/m$^2$ and 45–60 mg/m$^2$ were compared for late effects on contractility. Fewer children treated with 30 mg/m$^2$ had depressed contractility (9%, 6/65) than those treated with the higher dose (46%, 13/28) ($P < .001$). Thus, late depressed contractility in survivors of childhood ALL appears related to gender, as well as to the dose per cycle and the cumulative dosage of doxorubicin. These rela-

tionships are not well understood, but these factors should be considered in designing and conducting treatment protocols.

Elevated left ventricular afterload secondary to reduced left ventricular wall thickness is the most common late cardiac effect of doxorubicin therapy for childhood cancer and results in depressed left ventricular performance [4]. Chronically elevated afterload may be deleterious to long-term left ventricular contractility [70]. Progressive abnormal elevation of afterload occurs in the majority of patients. Late congestive heart failure, high-grade ectopy, and sudden death have been noted in some of the patients we follow who have elevated afterload and depressed left ventricular function. We assessed the long-term serial effects of afterload reduction with enalapril on left ventricular loading conditions and function [31]. Sixteen patients who had received a mean of 413 mg/m$^2$ of doxorubicin for childhood cancer diagnosed at a mean age of 8.7 years were treated with enalapril 7.2 years after completion of doxorubicin for elevated left ventricular afterload, defined as a mean end-systolic wall stress = 105 ± 22 g/cm$^2$ (normal = 40 to 60 g/cm$^2$). Eight asymptomatic patients (50%) had moderate to severe left ventricular dysfunction, and eight had congestive heart failure when enalapril began. Serial elevation of afterload from 73 to 105 g/cm$^2$ was noted during the 2.4 years before initiating enalapril and was accompanied by a reduction in both left ventricular contractility (stress–velocity index = -1.34 to -2.42 SD) and left ventricular performance (fractional shortening = 25% to 18%). During enalapril therapy, no patient had an adverse drug reaction, and afterload approached normal in all but one patient. By 0.4 years after initiation of enalapril, afterload had fallen to 74 ± 23 g/cm$^2$, contractility showed no further deterioration (-2.56 SD), and fractional shortening improved (23%) without a significant change in systolic or diastolic blood pressure. A later follow-up 1.9 years after the initiation of enalapril demonstrated that this improvement in left ventricular afterload and performance was sustained and was accompanied by preservation of contractility (afterload = 74 g/cm$^2$, contractility = 2.19 SD, fractional shortening = 23%).

In summary, enalapril therapy in doxorubicin-treated survivors of childhood cancer with abnormal left ventricular function and afterload appears safe and effective during the first 2 years of therapy. Therapy with enalapril results in a sustained reduction of left ventricular afterload and an improvement of left ventricular performance. However, a prospective study of enalapril therapy in doxorubicin-treated survivors of childhood cancer with abnormal left ventricular function or loading conditions is warranted to determine whether the course of late cardiotoxicity is altered.

## ARRHYTHMIAS

We have found ventricular tachycardia in 5% of survivors of childhood cancer at our institution an average of 7 years after completing anthracycline therapy [30]. These patients generally had significant left ventricular dysfunction due to depressed contractility or elevated afterload. Practically all of them had or developed chronic congestive heart failure within the subsequent 2 years. The use of 24-hour Holter monitoring of heart rhythm has been the most common way to detect these important late effects of therapy. Monitoring is particularly important in these patients, who have a higher incidence of sudden unexpected death than the general population, and thereby permits earlier invasive cardiac evaluation and therapy.

An increased frequency of QT$_c$ prolongation, supraventricular premature beats, supraventricular tachycardia, ventricular premature beats, couplets, and ventricular tachycardia were noted as late findings on electrocardiographic monitoring of long-term survivors of childhood cancer when compared with an age-matched healthy population [9]. These late findings confirm those noted at our institution and strengthen our recommendation for routine late monitoring of cardiac rate and rhythm.

## CONCLUSION

It is important for the following reasons not to rely exclusively on fractional shortening to determine the cardiac status in children treated for cancer: (1) Fractional shortening may not reveal all cases of cardiomyopathy; (2) it may not predict long-term cardiac outcome; and (3) it may not predict the response to cardiac therapy. The clinical implications of using fractional shortening as a measure of contractility in children without clinically apparent heart disease are many. Its usage may result in a misunderstanding of the incidence and course of cardiac involvement, may cause potentially harmful cardiac effects as a result of inappropriate therapy, and may lead to the denial of potential therapeutic interventions, among other problems.

Data upon which risk–benefit decisions regarding the early termination or modification of the anticancer regimen can be based are needed. We are concerned that clinicians may be placed in an uncomfortable medicolegal position by published but unproven recommendations to modify therapy when abnormalities are detected on invalidated cardiac studies obtained during acute therapy for childhood cancer. At this time, we suggest that (1) the data are insufficient to determine whether a modification of the anthracycline dosage based on cardiac monitoring does more harm than good, (2) none of the methods of screening for cardiac injury has been shown to be adequately predictive of late outcome, (3) the studies that have been done to evaluate the clinical utility of cardiac monitoring programs have failed to address adequately whether the ultimate outcome is improved and whether the results of selective dosage modification based on these indices are better than with arbitrary dosage limits without cardiac monitoring, and (4) the adoption of recommendations for screening and modification would inhibit the determination of whether the recommended screening program is truly effective. Routine monitoring of long-term survivors, however, is encouraged.

## ACKNOWLEDGMENTS

The authors thank Cynthia Barber for her editorial suggestions. This work was supported in part by grants CA34183, CA06516, and RO1HL48012-01 from the National Institutes of Health and a Clinical Investigator Award of the National Heart, Lung and Blood Institute of the National Institutes of Health, Bethesda, Maryland (HL01816).

## REFERENCES

1. Minow RA, Benjamin RS, Gottlieb JA: Adriamycin (NSC-123127) cardiomyopathy—an overview with determination of risk factors. Cancer Chemother Rep (pt 3) 6:195–201, 1975.
2. Hausdorf G, Mork G, Beron G, Erttmann R, Winkler K, Landbeck G, Keck EW: Long-term doxorubicin cardiotoxicity in childhood: Noninvasive evaluation of the contractile state and diastolic filling. Br Heart J 60:309–315, 1988.
3. Goorin AM, Chauvenet AR, Perez-Atayde AR, Cruz J, McKone R, Lipshultz SE: Initial congestive heart failure, six to ten years after doxorubicin chemotherapy for childhood cancer. J Pediatr 116:144–147, 1990.
4. Lipshultz SE, Colan SD, Gelber RD, Perez-Atayde AR, Sallan SE, Sanders SP: Late cardiac effects of doxorubicin therapy for acute lymphoblastic leukemia in childhood. N Engl J Med 324:808–815, 1991.
5. Yeung ST, Yoong C, Spink J, Galbraith A, Smith PJ: Functional myocardial impairment in children treated with anthracyclines for cancer. Lancet 337:816–818, 1991.
6. Weesner KM, Bledsoe M, Chauvenet A, Wofford M: Exercise echocardiography in the detection of anthracycline cardiotoxicity. Cancer 68:435–438, 1991.
7. Steinherz LJ, Steinherz PG, Tan CTC, Heller G, Murphy L: Cardiac toxicity 4 to 20 years after completing anthracycline therapy. J Am Med Assoc 266:1672–1677, 1991.
8. Klewer SE, Goldberg SJ, Donnerstein RL, Berg RA, Hutter JJ: Dobutamine stress echocardiography: A sensitive indicator of diminished myocardial function in asymptomatic doxorubicin-treated long-term survivors of childhood cancer. J Am Coll Cardiol 19:394–400, 1992.
9. Larsen RL, Jakacki RI, Vetter VL, Meadows AT, Silber JH, Barber G: Electrocardiographic changes and arrhythmias after cancer therapy in children and young adults. Am J Cardiol 70:73–77, 1992.
10. Anonymous: Childhood cancer, anthracyclines, and the heart. Lancet 339:1388–1389, 1992.
11. Meadows AT, Krejmas NL, Belasco JB: The medical cost of cure: Sequelae in survivors of childhood cancer. In Van Eys J, Sullivan MP (eds): Status of the Curability of Childhood Cancers. New York: Raven Press, 1980, pp 263–276.
12. Pediatric Oncology Group. Progress against childhood cancer: The Pediatric Oncology Group experience. Pediatrics 89:597–600, 1992.
13. Mandelson MT, Li FP: Survival of children with cancer. J Am Med Assoc 255:1572, 1986.
14. Blatt J, Bleyer WA: Late effects of childhood cancer and its treatment. In Pizzo PA, Poplack DG (eds): Principles and Practice of Pediatric Oncology. Philadelphia: J.B. Lippincott, 1989, pp 1003–1025.
15. Ross J Jr: Control of cardiac performance. In Berne RM, Sperelakis N, Geiger SR (eds): Handbook of Physiology: The Cardiovascular System, vol 1. Baltimore: Williams & Wilkins, 1979, pp 533–580.
16. Ross J Jr: Afterload mismatch and preload reserve: A conceptual framework for the analysis of ventricular function. Prog Cardiovasc Dis 18:255–264, 1976.
17. Weber KT, Janicki JS: The heart as a muscle-pump system and the concept of heart failure. Am Heart J 98:371–384, 1979.
18. Borow KM: Clinical assessment of contractility in the symmetrically contracting left ventricle. Mod Concepts Cardiovasc Dis 57:29–34, 1988.
19. Parmley WW: Pathophysiology and current

therapy of congestive heart failure. J Am Coll Cardiol 13:771–785, 1989.

20. Peterson KL, Skloven D, Ludbrook P, Uther JB, Ross J Jr: Comparison of isovolumic and ejection phase indices of myocardial performance in man. Circulation 49:1088–1101, 1974.

21. Colan SD, Borow KM, Neumann A: Left ventricular end-systolic wall stress-velocity of fiber shortening relation: A load-independent index of myocardial contractility. J Am Coll Cardiol 4:715–724, 1984.

22. Kass DA, Maughan LW, Zhong MG, Kono A, Sunagawa K, Sagawa K: Comparative influence of load versus inotropic state on indexes of ventricular contractility: Experimental and theoretical analysis based on pressure–volume relationships. Circulation 76:1422–1436, 1987.

23. Borow KM, Lang RM, Neumann A, Carroll JD, Rajfer SI: Physiologic mechanisms governing hemodynamic responses to positive inotropic therapy in patients with dilated cardiomyopathy. Circulation 77:625–637, 1988.

24. Gleason WL, Braunwald E: Studies on the first derivative of the ventricular pressure pulse in man. J Clin Invest 41:80–91, 1962.

25. Krayenbuehl HP, Rutishauser W, Wirz P, Amende I, Mehmel H: High fidelity left ventricular pressure measurements of the assessment of cardiac contractility in man. Am J Cardiol 31:415–427, 1973.

26. Larsen RL, Barber G, Heise CT, August CS: Exercise assessment of cardiac function in children and young adults before and after bone marrow transplantation. Pediatrics 89:722–729, 1992.

27. Colan SD, Parness IA, Spevak PJ, Sanders SP: Development modulation of myocardial mechanics: Age- and growth-related alterations in afterload and contractility. J Am Coll Cardiol 19:619–629, 1992.

28. Lipshultz SE, Colan SD, Sanders SP, Sallan SE: Cardiac mechanics after growth hormone therapy in pediatric adriamycin recipients. Pediatr Res 25:153A (abstr), 1989.

29. Lipshultz SE, Colan SD, Sanders SP, Perez-Atayde A, Sallan SE: Late myocardial growth impairment in children treated with Adriamycin (adr). Am J Cardiol 64:416 (abstr), 1989.

30. Lipshultz SE, Colan SD, Walsh EP, Sanders SP, Sallan SE: Ventricular tachycardia and sudden unexplained death in late survivors of childhood malignancy treated with doxorubicin. Pediatr Res 27:145A (abstr), 1990.

31. Lipshultz SE, Colan SD, Mone SM, Sallan SE, Gelber RD, Sanders SP: Afterload reduction therapy in long term survivors of childhood cancer treated with doxorubicin. Circulation 84:II-659 (abstr), 1991.

32. Lipshultz SE, Colan SD, Gelber RD, Mone SM, Sanders SP, Sallan SE: The effects of gender and doxorubicin dose rate on left ventricular contractility in late survivors of childhood leukemia. Circulation 86:I-363 (abstr), 1992.

33. Borow KM, Neumann A, Marcus RH, Sareli P, Lang RM: Effects of simultaneous alterations in preload and afterload on measurements of left ventricular contractility in patients with dilated cardiomyopathy: Comparisons of ejection phase, isovolumetric and end-systolic force–velocity indexes. J Am Coll Cardiol 20:787–795, 1992.

34. Ricci DR: Afterload mismatch and preload reserve in chronic aortic regurgitation. Circulation 66:826–834, 1982.

35. Wisenbaugh T, Booth D, DeMaria A, Nissen S, Waters J: Relationship of contractile state to ejection performance in patients with chronic aortic valve disease. Circulation 73:47–53, 1986.

36. Wisenbaugh T, Spann JF, Carabello BA: Differences in myocardial performance and load between patients with similar amounts of chronic aortic versus chronic mitral regurgitation. J Am Coll Cardiol 3:916–923, 1984.

37. Zile MR, Gaasch WH, Levine HJ: Left ventricular stress-dimension-shortening relations before and after correction of chronic aortic and mitral regurgitation. Am J Cardiol 56:99–105, 1985.

38. Dorn GW, Donner R, Assey ME, Spann JF, Wiles HB, Carabello BA: Alterations in left ventricular geometry, wall stress, and ejection performance after correction of congenital aortic stenosis. Circulation 78:1358–1364, 1988.

39. Colan SD, Sanders SP, Inglefinger JR, Harmon W: Left ventricular mechanics and contractile state in children and young adults with end-stage renal disease: Effect of dialysis and renal transplantation. J Am Coll Cardiol 10:1085–1094, 1987.

40. Colan SD: Assessment of ventricular and myocardial performance. In Fyler DC (ed): Nadas' Pediatric Cardiology. Philadelphia: Hanley & Belfus, 1992, pp 225–248.

41. Lipshultz SE, Orav EJ, Sanders SP, Rubin AH, McIntosh K, Colan SD: Abnormal cardiac structure and function in HIV-infected children treated with zidovudine. N Engl J Med 327:1260–1265, 1992.

42. Taliercio CP, Seward JB, Driscoll DJ, Fisher LD, Gersch BJ, Tajik AJ: Idiopathic dilated cardiomyopathy in the young: Clinical profile and natural history. J Am Coll Cardiol 6:1126–1131, 1985.

43. Griffin ML, Hernandez A, Martin TC, Goldring D, Bolman RM, Spray TL, Strauss AW: Dilated cardiomyopathy in infants and children. J Am

Coll Cardiol 11:139–144, 1988.

44. Unverferth DV, Magorien RD, Moeschberger ML, Baker PB, Fetters JK, Leier CV: Factors influencing the one-year mortality of dilated cardiomyopathy. Am J Cardiol 54:147–152, 1984.

45. Massie BM, Conway M: Survival of patients with congestive heart failure: Past, present and future prospects. Circulation 75:IV-11–19, 1987.

46. Lipshultz SE, Sanders SP, Colan SD, Orav EJ, McIntosh K: The use of left ventricular fractional shortening as an index of contractility in HIV-infected children. Am J Cardiol 66:521 (abstr), 1990.

47. Lipshultz SE, Orav EJ, Sanders SP, McIntosh K, Colan SD: Limitation of fractional shortening as an index of contractility in HIV-infected children. (Submitted).

48. Packer M, Carver JR, Rodeheffer RJ, et al.: Effect of oral milrinone on mortality in severe chronic heart failure. N Engl J Med 325:1468–1475, 1991.

49. Echt DS, Liebson PR, Mitchell LB, et al.: Mortality and morbidity in patients receiving encainide, flecainide, or placebo—the cardial arrhythmia suppression trial. N Engl J Med 324:781–787, 1991.

50. Henderson IC, Sloss LJ, Jaffe N, Blum RH, Frei E: Serial studies of cardiac function in patients receiving Adriamycin. Cancer Treat Rep 62:923–929, 1978.

51. Henderson IC, Frei E: Adriamycin and the heart. N Engl J Med 300:310–311, 1979.

52. Colan SD, Sanders SP, Borow KM: Physiologic hypertrophy: Effects on left ventricular systolic mechanics in athletes. J Am Coll Cardiol 9:776–783, 1987.

53. Steinherz LJ, Grahm T, Hurwitz R, Sondheimer HM, Schwartz RG, Shaffer EM, Sandor G, Benson L, Williams R: Guidelines for cardiac monitoring of children during and after anthracycline therapy: Report of the cardiology committee of the Children's Cancer Study Group. Pediatrics 89:942–949, 1992.

54. Gilladoga AC, Manuel C, Tan CTC, Wollner N, Sternberg SS, Murphy ML: The cardiotoxicity of Adriamycin and daunomycin in children. Cancer 37:1070–1078, 1976.

55. Lefrak EA, Pitha J, Rosenheim S, Gottlieb JA: A clinicopathologic analysis of Adriamycin cardiotoxicity. Cancer 32:302–314, 1973.

56. Tan C, Etcubanas E, Wollner N, et al.: Adriamycin: An antitumor antibiotic in the treatment of neoplastic diseases. Cancer 32:9–17, 1973.

57. Van Hoff DD, Rozencweig M, Layard M, et al.: Daunomycin-induced cardiotoxicity in children and adults. Am J Med 62:200–208, 1977.

58. Bender KS, Shematck JP, Leventhal BG, Kan JS: QT interval prolongation associated with anthracycline cardiotoxicity. J Pediatr 105:442–444, 1984.

59. Schwartz CL, Hobbie WL, Truesdell SC, Constine LS, Clark EB: QTc prolongation in anthracycline treated survivors of childhood cancer. Proc Am Soc Clin Oncol 9:292 (abstr), 1990.

60. Tamminga RYJ, Bink-Boelkens MThE, Kievit J: Ventricular late potentials: Another expression of cardiotoxicity of cystostatic drugs in children? Int J Cardiol 36:283–288, 1992.

61. Borow KM, Henderson IC, Neuman A, Colan S, Grady S, Papish S, Goorin A: Assessment of left ventricular contractility in patients receiving doxorubicin. Ann Intern Med 99:750–756, 1983.

62. Glamann DB, Lange RA, Corbett JR, Hillis LD: Utility of various radionuclide techniques for distinguishing ischemic from nonischemic dilated cardiomyopathy. Arch Intern Med 152:769–772, 1992.

63. McKillop JH, Bristow MR, Goris ML, Billingham ME, Bockemuehl K: Sensitivity and specificity of radionuclide ejection fractions in doxorubicin cardiotoxicity. Am Heart J 106:1048–1056, 1983.

64. Parrish MD, Boucek RJ, Burger J, Artman MF, Partain CL, Graham TP: Exercise radionuclide ventriculography in children: Normal values for exercise variables and right and left ventricular function. Br Heart J 54:509–516, 1985.

65. Dreyer Z, Mahoney DH, Steuber CP, Guidry G, Hillman K, Lacy J: Tantalum 178 cardiac imaging childhood cancer survivors: Complete evaluation in a single heartbeat. Proc Am Soc Ped Hem Oncol 1:16 (abstr), 1992.

66. Billingham ME, Bristow MR: Evaluation of anthracycline cardiotoxicity: Predictive ability and functional correlation of endomyocardial biopsy. In Proceedings of the Workshop on Mitoxantrone Cardiotoxicity and the Workshop on Clinical Evaluation of Anthracycline Cardiotoxicity. Cancer treatment symposia, vol 3. Washington, DC: Government Printing Office, NIH publ no 84-2690, 1984, pp 71–76.

67. Isner JM, Ferrans, VJ, Cohen SR, et al.: Clinical and morphologic cardiac findings after anthracycline chemotherapy. Am J Cardiol 51:1167–1174, 1983.

68. Sallan SE, Clavell LA: Cardiac effects of anthracyclines used in the treatment of childhood acute lymphoblastic leukemia: A 10 year experience. Sem Oncol 11:19–21, 1984.

69. Sallan SE: Personal communication, 1992.

70. Borow KM, Colan SD, Neumann A: Altered left ventricular mechanics in patients with valvular aortic stenosis and coarctation of the aorta: Effects on systolic performance and late outcome. Circulation 72:515–522, 1985.

# 7. Anthracycline-Related Cardiac Damage

Laurel J. Steinherz, M.D., Peter G. Steinherz, M.D., and Glenn Heller, Ph.D.

The anthracyclines are among the most useful antineoplastic agents. However, their use is limited by a toxic cardiomyopathy resulting in myocyte damage with acute, subacute, and chronic manifestations [1–3]. The acute symptoms closely follow a dose and can involve dysrhythmia, pericardial effusion, and acute decrease in contractility with resultant cardiac failure [4]. The subacute clinical manifestations can occur from days to up to 2 years after the last dose, with a peak onset of cardiac failure at 1–3 months after cessation of therapy [3,5]. Serial myocardial biopsy, during chemotherapy, has demonstrated that there is a linear increase in structural damage to the myocardium, with increasing cumulative dose [6]. By contrast, there is an exponential increase in deterioration of cardiac function with increasing cumulative dose [3,5]. There is also enhancement of cardiac toxicity by mediastinal irradiation [7,8].

Initially, attempts to avoid toxicity have depended upon an arbitrary imposition of a peak "safe" total cumulative dose [9]. However, there is considerable variation in individual susceptibility, hence some patients develop cardiac failure at doses within the accepted safe range [5]. More recent attempts to prevent toxicity have included alterations of dose schedules to decrease peak blood concentrations. Weekly dosage schedules and continuous infusion of the anthracyclines have been used for this purpose [10,11]. There have been periodic attempts to use protective agents [12], and to develop less toxic analogs. Dose adjustment, guided by serial noninvasive monitoring of patients with echocardiography and radionuclide cardiac cineangiography (RNCA), has reduced early clinical symptoms [13,14]. However, subclinical structural damage is still produced. In recent years, intensive management of symptomatic patients has improved early symptoms and stabilized most patients. Early studies such as that of Dresdale et al. [15], evaluating patients up to 4 years post-doxorubicin adjuvant chemotherapy, suggested that cardiac performance actually improved with time.

However, we had noted by 1980 decreasing contractility measurements after 6 or more years of follow-up in two of our patients who had suffered cardiac failure at the end of anthracycline therapy. These patients had exhibited initial improvement over the first 5 years of the posttherapy period [16,17], similar to that described by Dresdale et al. Both of our patients had been able to discontinue their cardiac medication transiently by 5 years postanthracycline, but both later became dependent on them again. We surmised that patients who never developed early congestive heart failure but had subclinical myocardial damage could be similarly affected. Therefore, we began a combined retrospective and prospective study of the

*Cardiac Toxicity After Treatment for Childhood Cancer*, pages 63–72, ©1993 Wiley-Liss, Inc.

cardiac function of patients after anthracycline therapy.

## PATIENTS AND METHODS

All patients who had completed chemotherapy and were free of recurrence for 4 years were eligible for the study, and for cardiac evaluation during their routine general follow-up evaluation. In addition, the pediatric oncologists were encouraged to plan future cardiac evaluations for their ongoing patients upon reaching the point of 5 years after discontinuation of therapy. Periodic evaluations were to be obtained thereafter as long as possible, until further predictive information became available to define an endpoint, if any. The study was limited to patients who had received $\geq 200$ mg/m$^2$ of doxorubicin and/or daunorubicin and were off therapy and free of malignant disease for at least 4 years. Patients treated with other known cardiotoxic agents such as AMSA (4'-(9-Acridinylamino)methanesulfon-m-anisidide) and deoxycoformycin were excluded. The results of the first 100 patients studied were presented at the 3rd World Congress of Pediatric Cardiology in June of 1985 [17], and a more extensive analysis of 201 patients was presented at the American Society of Clinical Oncology in 1989 and has recently been published [18].

Sixty-nine patients have since been added, forming a database of 270 patients for the present updated study. The patients were 2–23 years of age, with a median of 10 years of age at the end of therapy. They had received a total cumulative anthracycline dose of 200–1,275 mg/m$^2$, median 435 mg/m$^2$, by bolus or rapid infusion using an intermittent daily × 3 treatment schedule. Seventy patients (26%) had received a total dose of $\geq 500$ mg/m$^2$, and 75 had received mediastinal radiotherapy.

The patients had been treated for leukemia or a solid tumor. The length of follow-up after completion of therapy was 4–21 years, median 8 years. Ninety-one patients were evaluated 10 or more years after completion of chemotherapy.

Two hundred sixty-nine patients had echocardiograms at the time of long-term follow-up evaluation, one had only an RNCA, and 37 had both RNCA and echocardiography performed. The determinations analyzed on echocardiography included left ventricular end-diastolic and end-systolic dimensions, fractional shortening (FS), and left and right systolic time-interval indices. The echocardiogram was considered abnormal if the fractional shortening was below 29% and abnormalities of the other determinations were used as confirmatory evidence. The RNCA was considered abnormal if the ejection fraction was below 50% or decreased with exercise. The scan was borderline if the ejection fraction was 50–55% and did not increase with stress. Eight patients had endomyocardial biopsy, one had examination of the heart at cardiac transplantation, and one had myocardial examination at autopsy. Ninety-five patients had echocardiograms documenting cardiac status during the year following the last dose of anthracycline.

Since all but one of the patients had echocardiograms and less than one-third had RNCA, the echocardiographic results were used for determination of cardiac status and analysis of risk factors. The RNCA results were used for confirmation of the echocardiographic findings and for determination of the status of the one patient without an echocardiogram.

## RESULTS

The results were analyzed to determine the incidence of abnormal cardiac function at long-term follow-up and the risk factors associated with increased cardio-toxicity. The overall incidence of abnormal cardiac status for the 270 patients was 21% (58/270). Thirty-four patients had mild cardiomyopathy (FS = 25–29%), 9 patients moderate (FS = 21–24%), and 15 patients had severe cardiomyopathy (FS = 11–20%).

The risk factors examined included age at end therapy, total cumulative dose received, mediastinal radiation, and length of follow-up. The age at end of therapy (reflecting the age during therapy) did not appear to be significantly related to the incidence of cardiotoxicity at long-term follow-up. The incidence of abnormality of fractional shortening on echocardiogram of the patients treated in their teens was similar to that of the patients treated at under 6 years of age, and even under 3 years of age.

There was a highly significant predictive correlation between the end-therapy echocardiogram and the late follow-up cardiac studies (Fig. 1). Seventy-nine of the 95 patients who had echocardiograms during the first year following completion of chemotherapy were documented to have normal echocardiograms at that time. Of these, 70/79 (89%) remained normal, with an 11% incidence of long-term abnormality for this group. This was markedly different from the patients with abnormal echocardiograms during the year after chemotherapy, who remained abnormal or even worsened in 69% of cases. Moreover, those patients who did have an abnormal fractional shortening at long-term follow-up, after having been normal 1 year after chemotherapy, were only mildly abnormal, except for two patients. By contrast, more than one-third of the patients with abnormal end-therapy echocardiograms had a severe abnormality of fractional shortening—specifically, 6/16 (38%) had a fractional shortening of

$\leq$20%. This difference could not be explained by differences of the other risk factors between the two groups. The median total cumulative anthracycline dose of the patients with normal end-therapy echocardiograms was 446 mg/m$^2$, and the median length of follow-up was 7 years. These are to be compared with a median total dose of 450 mg/m$^2$ for the patients with abnormal end-therapy echocardiograms and a median length of follow-up of 8 years.

Increased total cumulative dose received continued to correlate with an increased incidence of poor cardiac function at late testing (Fig. 2). Thirty-two of 200 (16%) of patients treated with <500 mg/m$^2$ were abnormal, compared with 26/70 (37%) of patients treated with $\geq$500 mg/m$^2$. The percent incidence of abnormality in patients who had received mediastinal irradiation was higher (25%) than those who did not (21%), and the incidence of abnormality in the patients who received $\geq$2,000cGy to the mediastinum was 32%.

There was a correlation between length of follow-up and an increasing incidence of abnormal cardiac studies. There was also an increase in the severity of the abnormality with time from completion of anthracycline therapy (Table 1). Twenty-six of 179 (15%) patients evaluated at 4–9 years postanthracycline, 23/72 (32%) of patients 10–14 years, and 9/19 (47%) of patients 15–20 years postanthracycline were abnormal.

The relationship between total dose and length of follow-up was examined to see if these were additive risk factors. We divided the group into low- and high-risk subgroups in terms of each risk factor. Total cumulative dose $\geq$500 mg/m$^2$ predicted more than twice the incidence of abnormality as dose <500 mg/m$^2$. Length of follow-up $\geq$10 years also predicted more

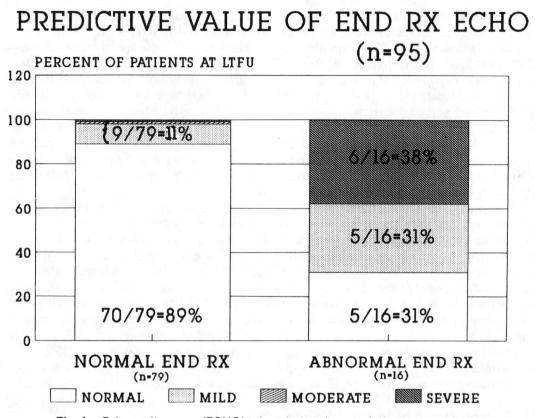

**Fig. 1.** Echocardiograms (ECHO) taken during the year following completion of anthracycline therapy (END RX) have prognostic implications for cardiac function at late cardiac follow-up (LTFU).

than twice the incidence of abnormality (35%), as did follow-up under 10 years (15%).

The whole group was further divided into three subgroups with none, one, or both of these risk factors. This identified the highest risk group as those with ≥500 mg/m² followed for ≥10 years. The incidence of abnormality in this group was 59%, approximately triple that of the other groups.

Multivariate analysis of the relationship between dose, length of follow-up, and mediastinal radiotherapy resulted in an equation that would predict the fractional shortening for a given total anthracycline dose and length of follow-up, with or with-

out radiotherapy, barring any other influence. The curves based on this equation (Fig. 3), with radiation on the left and without on the right, show a clear drop in the line of predicted FS for increasing years of follow-up between 5, 10, and 15 years. Clearly, many of our patients with severe compromise of contractility fall even below this prediction. The suboptimal fit of the data emphasizes that the equation ignores other important factors, including, notably, baseline and immediate posttherapy cardiac status. This information could not be included because it was available in less than half the patients, but, as demonstrated in Figure 1, they are powerful predictive factors.

# TOTAL CUMULATIVE DOSE

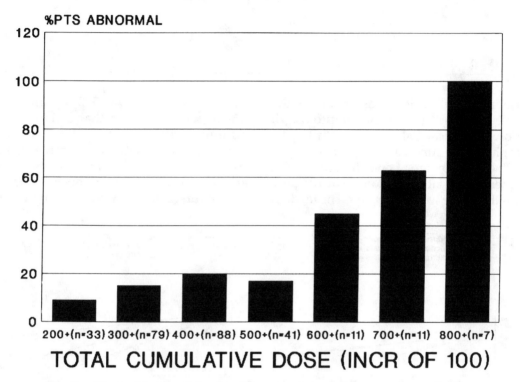

**%PTS ABNORMAL**

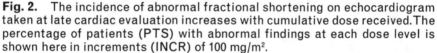

200+(n=33) 300+(n=79) 400+(n=88) 500+(n=41) 600+(n=11) 700+(n=11) 800+(n=7)

## TOTAL CUMULATIVE DOSE (INCR OF 100)

**Fig. 2.**   The incidence of abnormal fractional shortening on echocardiogram taken at late cardiac evaluation increases with cumulative dose received. The percentage of patients (PTS) with abnormal findings at each dose level is shown here in increments (INCR) of 100 mg/m².

## CLINICAL RELEVANCE

The clinical relevance of these abnormal long-term echocardiograms is apparent in 15 of the patients who developed late clinical symptoms simultaneous with echocardiographic deterioration. Thirteen patients had late cardiac failure and two had exertional dyspnea. All developed dysrhythmia and conduction abnormalities, and all 10 had fibrosis identified by pathological examination of the myocardium. Five of the patients had experienced cardiac symptoms the year after therapy, four requiring prolonged digoxin therapy,

and one requiring digoxin for only 1 month. All improved over the first 4 years, only to deteriorate 6–8 years postchemotherapy. Three died suddenly, with two patients having documented arrhythmia as a cause.

The 10 other patients had no early cardiac symptoms. Five had mildly abnormal "interim late" echocardiograms, and the others had no interim echocardiograms. All developed symptoms 8–19 years (median 14 years) postchemotherapy with severely abnormal cardiac function on echocardiogram, RNCA, and cardiac catheterization. They had similar abnormalities of conduction and rhythm. Six had

**TABLE 1.**

| Follow-Up Years | Mild | Moderate | Severe | Total No. Abnormal |
|---|---|---|---|---|
| 4–9 | 18/26 (70%) | 4/26 (15%) | 4/26 (15%) | 26 |
| 10–14 | 15/23 (65%) | 2/23 (9%) | 6/23 (26%) | 23 |
| 15–20 | 1/9 (11%) | 3/9 (33%) | 5/9 (56%) | 9 |

endomyocardial biopsy, as did one of the patients with early and late symptoms. All showed myocardial fibrosis with hypertrophy of the surviving myocytes.

The median age at end therapy for the patients with late symptoms was 10 years, and the range was 2–17 years. The median total dose received was 540 mg/m². Six patients were given less than 500 mg/m², and three less than 400 mg/m². The median time to the onset of late failure was 12 years, occurring earlier in patients with early failure and later in those without early failure. Nine patients had begun or

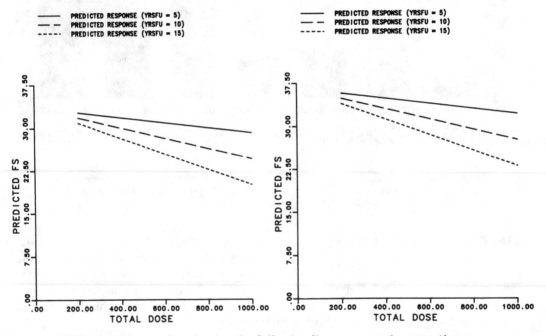

**Fig. 3.** Graphs produced using the following linear regression equation: FS = 36.65 - 3.04 (r) - .00091 (totdose) × (yrsfu) where r = 0 if the child received no mediastinal irradiation; where r = 1 if the child received mediastinal irradiation. (totdose) × (yrsfu) = the child's total cumulative dose multiplied by the number of years the child has been followed, and FS = the late echocardiogram fractional shortening predicted by the model. This demonstrates the negative effects of the product of total cumulative dose and years of follow-up (yrsfu) on fractional shortening at late echocardiogram. Decrements of fractional shortening between the 5-, 10-, and 15-year lines increase at higher total dose of anthracycline. The panel on the **left** is with mediastinal irradiation and the panel on the **right** is without mediastinal irradiation.

increased a recreational weight-lifting program or began heavy lifting at work during the months immediately preceding their late episode of pulmonary edema. Two of these patients were previously competitive track runners. Two other patients had begun using ethanol and/or cocaine just prior to congestive heart failure.

The patients were treated with digoxin, afterload-reducing agents including hydralazine and various angiotensin-converting enzyme inhibitors, and diuretics; those with symptomatic tachyrhythmias received antiarrhythmic agents. They have all responded to initial treatment of their late decompensation and have remained relatively stable for 1–9 years, median 3 years, in most cases resuming an active life. Only one patient ultimately succumbed to cardiac failure.

Arrhythmias, including complex ventricular tachyrhythmias, bradyarrhythmias, and conduction disturbances, have been a major problem in this group of patients. In addition to the three patients with sudden death, two patients had syncope, requiring cardiac transplant in one and an automatic implanted cardiac defibrillator in the second patient.

## DISCUSSION

Late abnormalities of cardiac function and rhythm have only recently been recognized as a significant problem in patients after successful completion of chemotherapy including anthracyclines. Since 1985, several studies have investigated the incidence [18–32], severity, and clinical significance of the problem. The incidence has varied greatly depending on the length of follow-up and the sensitivity of the methods of cardiac evaluation employed in each study. Techniques utilized have included history (at times by mailed survey), radiography, echocardiography, Doppler cardiography, RNCA, evaluation of

exercise hemodynamics and performance, challenge with pharmacologic afterload manipulation and dobutamine, electrocardiogram (ECG), continuous taped 24-hour ECG recordings, cardiac catheterization, intracardiac transcatheter electrophysiology, and endomyocardial biopsy. Within each technique there is a wide variation of sensitivity of testing parameters available. For example, echocardiography can define a simple fractional shortening or can explore indices of end-systolic wall stress compared to rate-corrected velocity of circumferential fiber shortening or indices of diastolic function, and can examine the response of all of these to exercise or pharmacological challenge as well. The analysis in this study by fractional shortening on resting echocardiography is relatively insensitive, and therefore must underestimate the extent of subclinical abnormal cardiac function. Consequently, the incidence of abnormality of 35% in the patients followed $\geq$10 years, including 24% of those treated with <500 mg/m$^2$, must be viewed as even more disquieting.

The present efforts at prevention through variation of anthracycline delivery schedule [10,11], monitoring of cardiac function during therapy, and, we hope, the eventual success of pretreatment with the cardioprotectant ADR529 (ICRF) [12] should reduce the scope of this problem in the future. In the meantime, we can expect that approximately 5% of patients treated with early regimens are at risk of developing symptomatic cardiac decompensation up to 20 years after discontinuation of chemotherapy. We do not know what the incidence will be with still longer follow-up. Treatment has involved established therapy of cardiac failure and arrhythmias as described above, and referral for cardiac transplantation when medical management was unsuccessful. In addition, we now attempt to counsel our patients who have even minimal evidence of cardiac dysfunction to avoid the lifestyle factors found to have been associated with the decompensation of the late symptomatic patients, such as immoderate intake of ethanol, cocaine and steroid abuse, and heavy vocational and recreational weight lifting. The coincidence of weight lifting to the time of decompensation in 9 of 15 of our patients may indicate that this is contraindicated in patients who have received anthracyclines. Evidence suggests that increased peripheral resistance during lifting causes increased cardiac work, higher wall stress, and decreased coronary artery flow [33,34]. It is known to contribute to myocardial hypertrophy [35]. It may produce a subclinical amount of subendocardial ischemia that may further injure the already scarred myocardium.

## CONCLUSION

This significant incidence of abnormal cardiac function on long-term follow-up noninvasive monitoring and the late symptomatic cardiac decompensation of 15 of our patients disproves the initial impression that anthracycline-induced cardiac damage will heal with long-lasting improvement of cardiac function. Although the majority of children who received anthracycline chemotherapy have no cardiac dysfunction on follow-up 4–21 years posttherapy, those patients with even mildly abnormal early echocardiogram, and especially those with early clinical symptoms, high cumulative dose, and mediastinal radiation, are at higher risk and may decompensate on longer follow-up. This is characterized by progressive echocardiographic and ECG abnormalities and worsening dysrhythmia. The pathology noted on late autopsy and on cardiac biopsy has been mainly cardiac fibro-sis with less prominent vacuolization than on biopsy during therapy.

The experience with some of our patients indicates that there is some risk for even the patients with no early symptoms. Of note, the median follow-up of our large series is still under 10 years, and the patients with no early symptoms decompensated after 14 years. Still longer follow-up of cardiac function and ECGs is recommended for these patients. It is our responsibility to continue to follow the cardiac status of our patients who received anthracyclines, both for their care and in order to plan better therapy for the future.

## REFERENCES

1. Tan C, Etcubans E, Wollner N, Rosen G, Gilladoga A, Showel J, Murphy ML, Krakoff IH: Adriamycin—an antitumor antibiotic in the treatment of neoplastic disease. Cancer 32:9–17, 1973.
2. Bristow MR, Billingham ME, Mason JW, Daniels JR: Clinical spectrum of anthracycline cardiotoxicity. Cancer Treat Rep 62:873–879, 1978.
3. Von Hoff DD, Rozencweig M, Layard M, et al.: Daunomycin-induced cardiotoxicity in children and adults. Am J Med 62:200–208, 1977.
4. Bristow MR, Thompson PD, Martin RP, et al.: Early anthracycline cardiotoxicity. Am J Med 65:823–832, 1978.
5. Von Hoff DD, Layard M, Basa P: Risk factors for doxorubicin induced congestive heart failure. Ann Intern Med 91:701–717, 1979.
6. Bristow MR: Pathophysiologic basis for cardiac monitoring in patients receiving anthracyclines. In ST Crook, SD Reich (eds): Anthracyclines: Current Status and New Developments. New York: Academic Press, 1980, pp 255–271.
7. Gilladoga AC, Manuel C, Tan CTC, Wollner N, Sternberg SS, Murphy ML: The cardiotoxicity of Adriamycin and daunomycin in children. Cancer 37:1070–1078, 1976.
8. Billingham ME, Bristow MR, Glastein E, Mason J, Masek M, Daniels J: Adriamycin cardiotoxicity: Endomyocardial biopsy evidence of enhancement by irradiation. Am J Surg Path 1:17–23, 1977.
9. Lefrak EA, Pitha J, Resenheim S, Gottlieb JA: A clinico-pathologic analysis of Adriamycin cardiotoxicity. Cancer 32:302–314, 1973.

10. Legha SS, Benjamin RS, Mackay B, et al.: Reduction of doxorubicin cardiotoxicity by prolonged continuous intravenous infusion. Ann Intern Med 96:133–138, 1982.

11. Torti FM, Bristow MR, Howes AE, et al.: Reduced cardiotoxicity of doxorubicin delivered on a weekly schedule: Assessment by endomyocardial biopsy. Ann Intern Med 99:745–749, 1983.

12. Speyer JL, Green MD, Kramer E, Rey M, Sanger J, Ward C, Dubin N, Ferrans V, Stecy P, Zeleniuch-Jacquotte A, Wernz J, Feit F, Slater W, Blum R, Muggia F: Protective effect of the bispiperazinedione ICRF 187 against doxorubucin-induced cardiac toxicity in women with advanced breast cancer. N Engl J Med 319:745–752, 1988.

13. Bloom K, Bini R, Williams C, et al.: Echocardiography in Adriamycin cardiotoxicity. Cancer 41:1265–1269, 1978.

14. Steinherz LJ, Graham T, Hurwitz R, Sandor G, Schwartz R, Shaffer E, Sondheimer H, Williams R: Guidelines for cardiac monitoring of children during and after anthracycline therapy. Report of the Cardiology Committee of the Children's Cancer Study Group. Pediatrics 89:942–949, 1992.

15. Dresdale A, Bonow R, Wesley R, Palmeri ST, Barr L, Mathison D, D'Angelo T, Rosenberg SA: Prospective evaluation of doxorubicin induced cardiomyopathy resulting from post surgical adjuvant treatment of patients with soft tissue sarcomas. Cancer 52:51–60, 1983.

16. Steinherz L, Murphy ML, Steinherz P, Rosen G, Robins J, Tan C: Cardiac function studies in children 4–11 years following cancer chemotherapy including anthracyclines. Proc Am Soc Clin Oncol 3:198, 1984 (abstr).

17. Steinherz L, Murphy ML, Steinherz P, Robins J, Tan C: Long-term cardiac followup 4–13 years post anthracycline therapy. In E Doyle, MA Engle, W Gersony, W Rashkin, N Talner (eds): Pediatric Cardiology. New York: Springer-Verlag, 1986, pp 1056–1061.

18. Steinherz LJ, Steinherz PG, Tan CTC, Heller G, Murphy ML: Cardiotoxicity 4–20 years after completing anthracycline therapy. J Am Med Assoc 266:1672–1677, 1991.

19. Steinherz LJ, Steinherz PG: Delayed anthracyclines cardiac toxicity. In VT DeVita, S Hellman, SA Rosenberg (eds): Cancer: Principles and Practice of Oncology. PPO Updates, vol 5, no 4, 1991, pp 1–15.

20. McDonald IG, Hobson ER: A comparison of the relative value of noninvasive techniques—echocardiography, systolic time intervals, and apex cardiography in the diagnosis of primary myocardial disease. Am Heart J 88:454–462, 1974.

21. Sutton GP, Stehman FB, Einhorn LH, Roth LM, Blessing JA, Ehrlich CE: Ten-year follow-up of patients receiving cisplatin, doxorubicin, and cyclophosphamide chemotherapy for advanced epithelial ovarian carcinoma. J Clin Oncol 7:223–229, 1989.

22. Mortensen S, Olsen H, Baandrup U: Chronic anthracycline cardiotoxicity: Hemodynamic and histopathological manifestations suggesting a restrictive endomyocardial disease. Br Heart J 55:274–282, 1986.

23. Hausdorf G, Morf G, Beron G, Erttmann R, Winkler K, Landbeck G, Keck EW: Long-term doxorubicin cardiotoxicity in childhood: Noninvasive evaluation of the contractile state and diastolic filling. Br Heart J 60:309–315, 1988.

24. Makinen L, Makipernaa A, Rautonen J, et al.: Long-term cardiac sequelae after treatment of malignant tumors with radiotherapy or cytostatics in childhood. Cancer 65:1913–1917, 1990.

25. Bigras J, Fournier A, Leclerc J, et al.: Study of the long term effects of anthracyclines on cardiac function. Proc Am Soc Ped Hem Oncol 3:19, 1990 (abstr).

26. LaMonte CS, Yeh SDJ, Straus DJ: Long-term follow-up of cardiac function in patients with Hodgkin's disease treated with mediastinal irradiation and combination chemotherapy including doxorubicin . Cancer Treat Rep 70:439–444, 1986.

27. Donaldson SS, Kaplan HS: Complications of treatment of Hodgkin's disease in children. Cancer Treat Rep 66:977–989, 1982.

28. Goorin AM, Chauvenet AR, Perez-Atayde AR, Cruz J, McKone R, Lipschultz SE: Initial congestive heart failure, six to ten years after doxorubicin chemotherapy for childhood cancer. J Pediatr 116:144–147, 1990.

29. Lipshultz SE, Colan SD, Gelber RD, Perez-Atayde AR, Sallen SA, Sanders SP: Late cardiac effects of doxorubicin in childhood lymphoblastic leukemia. N Engl J Med 324:808–815, 1991.

30. Weesner KM, Bledsoe M, Chauvenet A, Wofford M: Exercise echocardiography in the detection of anthracycline cardiotoxicity. Cancer 68:435–438, 1991.

31. Jakacki R, Silber J, Larsen R, Barber G, Goldwein J, Meadows A: Cardiac dysfunction following "low risk" cardiotoxic treatment for childhood malignancy. Pediatr Res 29:143A, 1991 (abstr).

32. Larsen RL, Barber G, Jakacki R, Silber J, Veller

VL, Meadows AT: Electrocardiographic changes and arrhythmias with anthracyclines and mediastinal irradiation. Am J Cardiol 70:73–77, 1992.

33. MacDougall JD, Tuxen D, Sale DG, Moroz JR, Sutton JR: Arterial blood pressure response to heavy resistance exercise. J Appl Phys 58:785–790, 1985.

34. Sullivan J, Hanson P, Rahko PS, Folts JD: Continuous measurement of left ventricular performance during and after maximal isometric deadlift exercise. Circulation 85:1406–1413, 1992.

35. Colan S, Sanders S, Borow K: Physiologic hypertrophy: Effects on left ventricular systolic mechanics in athletes. J Am Coll Cardiol 9:776–783, 1987.

# 8. Late Effects of Anthracycline Therapy in Childhood: Evaluation and Current Therapy

Gerd Hausdorf, M.D., Ph.D.

## CURRENT METHODS FOR THE EVALUATION OF CARDIAC FUNCTION

Evaluation of cardiac performance after anthracycline therapy in childhood includes a variety of methods, most of which focus solely on left ventricular function, while right ventricular function is usually neglected. The only exceptions are the endomyocardial biopsy [6–9], which is usually performed in the right ventricle, and right heart catheterization [10,11], which is routinely used for the evaluation of cardiac function and reserve in adults, but rarely in children. Right heart catheterization allows the assessment of the cardiac output, which reflects the function of the heart to act as a pump and its ability to maintain organ perfusion [10,11]. Additionally, the left ventricular filling pressure is assessed by measuring the "pulmonary wedge pressure" [11]. The latter gives an estimate for left ventricular function reflecting the left ventricular filling pressure necessary to maintain an adequate cardiac output [12,13]. However, endomyocardial biopsy and right heart catheterization are both invasive and potentially harmful. There is limited access to these methods, and they cannot regularly be performed serially. Although endomyocardial biopsy is an important diagnostic tool for acute anthracycline cardiotoxicity [6–10], its value for the evaluation of late damage is limited. Cardiac function seems to be of superior importance for the patient's quality of life in contrast to the histologic appearance of the myocardium [14].

The major advantage of radionuclide angiography is its independence of left ventricular geometry [3,5,11,15]. Most other methods used for the evaluation of cardiac function are dependent at least in part on ventricular geometry. Therefore the nuclear scan is an important diagnostic method for the evaluation of left ventricular function, which allows the analysis of ejection fraction and, depending on the equipment, of diastolic filling dynamics [15]. However, radionuclide angiography also has limitations. Myocardial wall thickness and consequently left ventricular wall stress cannot be evaluated by this method. The applicability of nuclear scans depends on the patient age, the resolution of the equipment used, and the skill of the investigator. The most important disadvantage is a substantial whole-body radiation dose, due to administration of a radionuclide. This is of particular concern in patients who previously received chemotherapy. Thus, radionuclide angiography should not be called a noninvasive method; it should not be performed serially because of the radiation exposure inherent to this method.

*Cardiac Toxicity After Treatment for Childhood Cancer*, pages 73–85, ©1993 Wiley-Liss, Inc.

In contrast to cardiac catheterization and radionuclide angiography, the echocardiographic methods (M-mode echocardiography, two-dimensional echocardiography, Doppler echocardiography) are clearly noninvasive, can be performed serially, and are inexpensive and available. Echocardiography allows the evaluation of left ventricular size and ejection fraction, as well as myocardial mass and wall thickness, both of which cannot be assessed by nuclear scans [16–24].

M-mode echocardiography, the standard method for the evaluation of left ventricular function, allows the exact and instantaneous evaluation of ventricular diameters, wall thicknesses, and left ventricular shortening [16–24]. Measuring fractional shortening, which is the percentage change of the left ventricular diameter during systole, is the standard parameter of systolic cardiac function. When the corresponding end-systolic blood pressure is measured simultaneously with the M-mode echocardiogram, end-systolic wall stress, which reflects left ventricular afterload, can be calculated from the left ventricular diameter, wall thickness, and end-systolic pressure [25–32]. Furthermore, when computer-assisted analysis of the instantaneous left ventricular dimension, posterior wall thickness, and their changes is performed, diastolic filling dynamics can be analyzed [33–36].

We conducted a study of late anthracycline cardiotoxicity performed 2 to 10 years after doxorubicin treatment (31–656 mg/m$^2$) using computer-assisted analysis of M-mode cumulative dosage echocardiograms [14]. An impairment of early diastolic function was found despite normal systolic function, the impairment of early diastolic function being related to the cumulative dose of doxorubicin (Fig. 1). Unfortunately, computer-assisted analysis of M-mode echocardiograms is rather time-consuming, not generally available, and dependent on the availability of a skilled investigator. There are, therefore, limitations to this sophisticated method for the serial evaluation of a large population.

In contrast to these limitations of the computer-assisted analysis of M-mode echocardiograms, Doppler echocardiography (pulsed Doppler) allows the evaluation of diastolic filling dynamics by the assessment of blood-flow velocities in a defined area of interest. Under the assumption of a laminar blood flow, these blood-flow velocities reflect the volume flow of blood. Rapid diastolic filling is reflected by the so-called "E-wave" of the blood flow through the mitral valve, while the so-called "A-wave" reflects the contraction. The ratio between the "E-wave" and the "A-wave" reflects the ratio between rapid and passive filling, being much easier to analyze using Doppler echocardiography than by the computer-assisted analysis of M-mode echocardiograms [37–39]. Additionally, stroke volume and cardiac index can be evaluated noninvasively using pulsed Doppler, limiting the need for invasive methods such as right heart catheterization, for the assessment of the cardiac index. As Doppler echocardiography is generally available, not time-consuming (for a well-trained investigator), and relatively inexpensive, it is an important method for the evaluation of late anthracycline cardiotoxicity.

While M-mode echocardiography is limited to the evaluation of one left ventricular diameter, two-dimensional echocardiography allows the evaluation of left ventricular geometry, regional wall motion, circumferential wall stress, and regional wall stresses [40–43]. Additionally, the left ventricular systolic and diastolic volumes can be estimated noninvasively. However, the evaluation of left ventricular volumes, geometry, regional wall motion, circumferential wall stress, and regional wall stress is time-consuming, dependent on the availability of a skilled investigator, not generally available, and of unknown

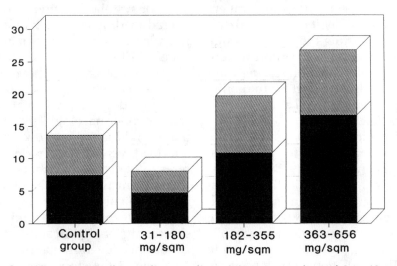

## Early Diastolic Filling and Cumulative Doxorubicin Dose (N = 55)

**Fig. 1.** When late anthracycline cardiotoxicity was evaluated 2 to 10 years after doxorubicin treatment (cumulative dose 31–656 mg/sqm) in childhood, computer-assisted analysis of M-mode echocardiograms showed a significant impairment of early diastolic function. The change of dimension between minimal left ventricular dimension and mitral valve opening increased significantly with increasing cumulative doxorubicin dose ($P < 0.0001$) [14].

clinical significance. Further studies will have to show if these methods are of additional value for the evaluation of late anthracycline cardiotoxicity.

Finally, nuclear magnetic resonance should be mentioned as a method for the assessment of cardiac function. Although this method is expensive and not generally available, it is noninvasive and allows the analyses of ventricular function, geometry, and wall thicknesses. Additionally, evaluation of blood flows is possible or will be possible soon. However, the future will have to show if this method can become a screening method for the serial evaluation of cardiac function.

## STRESS TESTING

Even when resting cardiac function is normal, "cardiac reserve" (the ability to increase cardiac function during exercise) can be abnormal. Therefore the sensitivity of the standard techniques mentioned above can be increased by stress testing. Two principal approaches to disclose reduced cardiac reserve are available: exercise testing and pharmacological "stress" testing. With exercise testing, either the ability to perform physical work or the ability to increase cardiac performance during stress is evaluated; several parameters such as maximal exercise capacity, maximal oxygen consumption, etc., which reflect the individual limitation to perform physical work, can be assessed [44–47]. Unfortunately, reduced exercise tolerance is not specific for reduced cardiac function [44,45].

However, its specifity can be increased if the ability to increase cardiac performance is evaluated during exercise [48]. Right heart catheterization, radionuclide angiography, or echocardiography can be performed at rest and during exercise to evaluate the ability to increase cardiac performance. While cardiac output is usually normal at resting conditions in compensated cardiomyopathy, it is abnormal during exercise, reflecting the cardiac limitation to perform exercise. Unfortunately, evaluating cardiac function during exercise depends, at least in part, on the ability to perform exercise, as well as on intrinsic cardiac function.

Pharmacological "stress testing" is an important new technique for the evaluation of cardiac function [49–58]. Increasing afterload pharmacologically using vasoactive drugs (methoxamine, phenylephrine, angiotensin) allows the evaluation of the left ventricular end-systolic stress-dimension and stress-shortening relations. These relations are "load-independent" measures of the contractile state, as they are (nearly) independent of preload and incorporating afterload. All the other parameters mentioned above are load-dependent; abnormal findings can be due either to abnormal loading conditions or an altered contractile state. From a methodologic point of view, only load-independent parameters should be used for the evaluation of systolic left ventricular function.

## EVALUATION OF SYSTOLIC FUNCTION: THEORETICAL AND PRACTICAL IMPLICATIONS

Systolic function is usually evaluated by the so-called "ejection-phase indices," such as fractional shortening, ejection fraction, mean fiber-shortening velocity, etc. These ejection-phase indices describe the ability of the heart to eject blood into the circulation. The change of diameter, area, or volume that occurs during systole is expressed as a percentage of the end-diastolic diameter, area, or volume. However, the ejection-phase indices are dependent on preload, afterload, heart rate, and the contractile state. This load dependency limits their diagnostic value for the evaluation of systolic function significantly, as altered loading conditions cannot be differentiated from an abnormal contractile state [49–58].

This is not only of theoretical importance, since ventricular shortening is significantly decreased when afterload is increased pharmacologically, even in normal individuals (Fig. 2). With increasing afterload, ventricular shortening deteriorates in patients with abnormal left ventricular function more significantly than in normal subjects. The slope of the relation between afterload and ventricular shortening is significantly steeper with abnormal left ventricular function (Fig. 3). Analysis of the slope of the relation between afterload and ventricular ejection or between afterload and end-systolic dimension has been shown to be (nearly) load-independent and highly sensitive to alterations of the contractile state [26,28,49–58].

Ventricular shortening

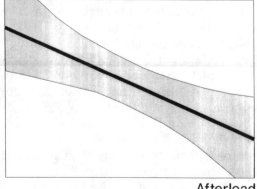

Afterload

**Fig. 2.** The figure shows schematically the relation between ventricular shortening and afterload. When afterload is increased pharmacologically, ventricular shortening decreases significantly in normal individuals.

## Ventricular shortening

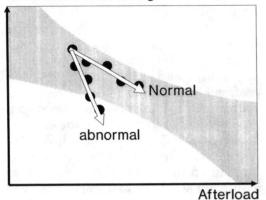

**Fig. 3.** The individual relations between ventricular shortening and afterload are shown for normal ventricular function and abnormal ventricular function schematically. When afterload is increased pharmacologically, the slope of the relation between afterload and ventricular shortening is significantly steeper with abnormal left ventricular function when compared with normal function.

However, the individual assessment of these relations cannot be applied as a screening method. It has been suggested that the analysis of ventricular ejection and the corresponding afterload at resting conditions could be of comparable diagnostic value and would simplify this approach significantly. To eliminate the influence of heart rate, the so-called "rate-corrected fiber-shortening velocity" was developed, which is the mean fiber-shortening velocity corrected for heart rate [57]. For the evaluation of systolic function, the data points for the "rate-corrected fiber-shortening velocity" and afterload are compared with the 95% confidence intervals of the relation between afterload and the "rate-corrected fiber-shortening velocity," assessed in normal subjects by pharmacological afterload increments [4,51,57].

The application of this approach for the relation between afterload and fractional shortening is shown schematically in Figure 4. Even if fractional shortening is reduced below normal, it can still be normal in relation to afterload. It has been argued that the contractile state would be normal as long as ventricular shortening related to afterload were within the normal range in Figure 4 [4,51,57]. However, this approach does not take into account the fact

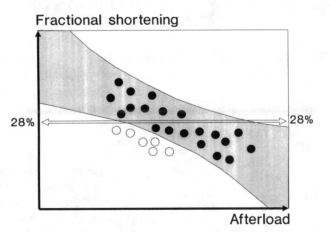

**Fig. 4** The relation between afterload and fractional shortening obtained by pharmacological afterload challenge in normal individuals is shown. Data points within this normal range are normal in respect to afterload, even when the fractional shortening is clearly reduced. Data points outside this normal range are abnormal.

that the relation between ejection and afterload is evaluated at resting conditions, while the normal range between afterload and ejection in Figure 4 has been evaluated during pharmacological afterload increments. Comparing data obtained at resting conditions with data obtained during a pharmacological intervention is methodologically incorrect [14,58]. Only data obtained under the same conditions can be compared.

Figure 5 shows the normal range for afterload and fractional shortening at resting conditions, and demonstrates that it is definitely abnormal for afterload to be increased at resting conditions. An increased afterload seems to be an early sign of anthracycline cardiotoxicity, as we showed in a previous study [14,51] (Fig. 6).

When late anthracycline cardiotoxicity was evaluated 2 to 10 years after doxorubicin treatment (cumulative dose 31–656 mg/m$^2$) in childhood, afterload was significantly increased despite normal fractional shortening, depending on the cumulative doxorubicin dose ($P < 0.03$). Sur-

prisingly, this was not shown for the pharmacological afterload challenge [14]. This has a simple explanation. Afterload in terms of end-systolic wall stress depends on the end-systolic pressure, left ventricular volume, and wall thickness. As left ventricular volume decreases toward end-systole and wall thickness increases concomitantly, the systolic wall stress is decreasing toward end-systole. Thus, end-systolic wall stress and afterload are dependent on the ability of the ventricle to reduce its size and to increase its wall thickness toward the end of systole. This ability to reduce its volume, increase its wall thickness, and thereby reduce its wall stress reflects the ability of the left ventricle to "unload itself" during ejection [55]. Thus, afterload is not a force or pressure the left ventricle has to overcome, but reflects the "unloading" of the left ventricle and thereby its contractile state. Therefore, afterload itself is a parameter of systolic function, indicating impaired "unloading" as a sensitive parameter of early left ventricular dysfunction.

## Fractional shortening

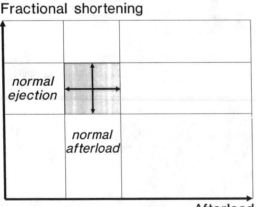

**Fig. 5.** The normal range for both fractional shortening and afterload is shown at resting conditions. At resting conditions the normal fractional shortening is 34 ± 10%, while the end-systolic stress (afterload) is 50 ± 10 g/sqm. An afterload above 70 g/sqm is abnormal.

## EVALUATION OF DIASTOLIC FUNCTION

Although dilative cardiomyopathy is basically characterized by systolic dysfunction, diastolic dysfunction occurs in the course of anthracycline cardiomyopathy [59]. Diastolic filling can be divided into three phases: relaxation, elastic recoil, and passive diastolic filling (Fig. 7). Relaxation is an active process, which reflects the unbinding between actin and myosin filaments, and is reflected by the "time constant of isovolumic pressure decay," which is measured before the mitral valve opens and diastolic filling starts. The next phase is called "elastic recoil," which is due to the elastic forces "stored" within the myocardium during contraction. Finally, passive diastolic filling occurs, which

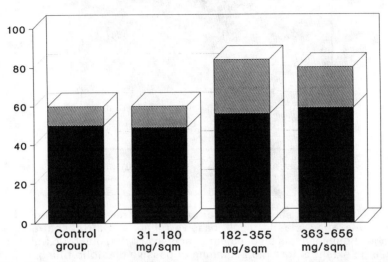

**Fig. 6.** When late anthracycline cardiotoxicity was evaluated 2 to 10 years after doxorubicin treatment (cumulative dose 31–656 mg/sqm) in childhood, afterload (at resting conditions) was significantly increased despite normal fractional shortening, depending on the cumulative doxorubicin dose ($P <$ 0.03) [14].

is due to the interaction of the elastic and viscoelastic properties of the myocardium and the filling pressure [60–62]. Passive filling is augmented by atrial contraction.

It seems to be important that diastolic filling occurs to a large extent during early diastole (Fig. 7), being affected by relaxation and elastic recoil. As elastic recoil depends on the preceding systole, early diastolic filling is at least in part dependent on systolic function. This is of particular importance, as early diastolic filling is an important and sensitive index for the evaluation of altered diastolic function, which can be assessed noninvasively by M-mode and Doppler echocardiography.

## CRITERIA FOR EVALUATION OF CARDIAC PERFORMANCE

Which parameters should be selected for the evaluation of late anthracycline cardiotoxicity? Although the sophisticated methods mentioned above are of great interest to cardiologists, they are usually time-consuming, not generally available, and not applicable for serial investigations in a large population. Additionally, little is known about the clinical relevance of these parameters.

The methods used for the serial evaluation of a large population have to fulfill the following criteria: They have to be noninvasive, generally available, relatively inexpensive, applicable in children and adults independent of age, without need for cooperation, and sensitive for the detection of impaired cardiac function. Additionally, these methods should be selected according to their clinical and therapeutic implications. To fulfill these criteria, the following investigations are selected for the evaluation of late anthracycline cardiotoxicity.

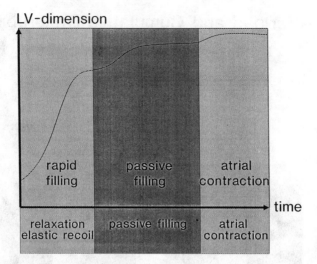

**Fig. 7.** The figure shows schematically the different phases of diastolic filling: relaxation, elastic recoil, passive filling, and atrial contraction. The change of dimension is also indicated and shows that diastolic filling occurs to a large extent before the beginning of passive diastolic filling, indicating the importance of "early" or "rapid" diastolic filling.

## Clinical Investigation

Clinical examination including careful history of exercise intolerance, heart failure, or arrhythmias is of great importance for clinical decisions that require differentiation between asymptomatic and symptomatic cardiac dysfunction.

## Echocardiographic Evaluation

Echocardiographic examination appears to be the most important, sensitive, and specific method for the detection of late anthracycline cardiotoxicity. Within the wide range of sophisticated methods, the following parameters should be assessed:

*End-diastolic diameter*, which indicates ventricular dilatation in dilative cardiomyopathy.

*Ventricular shortening* (fractional shortening, mean fiber shortening velocity, "rate-corrected fiber-shortening velocity"), which indicates reduced ventricular function in overt dilative cardiomyopathy.

*Afterload* (end-systolic wall stress), which reflects impaired "unloading" of the ventricle. Even when ventricular shortening is still within the normal range, afterload already can be abnormal.

*Diastolic filling* by evaluation of the E-/A-wave ratio using Doppler echocardiography, because impaired early diastolic filling seems to be an early and sensitive parameter of anthracycline cardiotoxicity.

The *cardiac index* (using Doppler echocardiography) should be analyzed in relation to the end-diastolic diameter of the left ventricle, because the cardiac index is usually kept in a normal range by increasing preload.

## Nuclear Scan (Optional)

Nuclear scans have the major advantage of being independent of left ventricular geometry and are useful to control echocardiographic measurements, but there is substantial whole-body radiation associated with this technique. Therefore the method should be considered optional and should not be performed serially in patients who already received chemotherapy. However, nuclear scans should be performed when echocardiography is impossible because of technical reasons.

## Electrocardiogram and Holter Monitoring

The sensitivity and specifity of electrocardiographic changes for late anthracycline-induced cardiotoxicity seems to be low. It is, however, the only method to detect disturbances of conduction, and repolarization, and to measure the QT interval. Additionally, Holter monitoring is the only method for the detection of arrhythmias, which are of significant clinical importance. As these investigations are easily performed, they should be included in the serial examination of these patients despite a low sensitivity and specificity.

## THERAPEUTIC IMPLICATIONS AND STRATEGIES

There is increasing evidence that the incidence of late anthracycline cardiotoxicity is much higher than assumed before [3–5,14,51]. There is still controversy about the evaluation of late anthracycline cardiotoxicity. Efforts should nonetheless focus not only on a concept for the serial evaluation of this disease but also on therapeutic strategies for patients who are at risk of developing progressive cardiac dysfunction leading to dilative cardiomyopathy. Little is known about the natural course of anthracycline cardiotoxicity. Despite this, some therapeutic suggestions can be made.

## Asymptomatic, Minimal Changes

Asymptomatic patients with borderline or minimal changes of cardiac function or with abnormalities of "sophisticated" parameters (as early diastolic filling) need no therapy because the clinical impact of these parameters is unknown. However, cardiac function should be monitored closely to detect any deterioration of cardiac performance.

## Asymptomatic, Increased Afterload

If the patient is asymptomatic and cardiac dysfunction is reflected only by an increased afterload (end-systolic wall stress >70 gm/cm$^2$), pharmacological afterload reduction using captopril or enalapril seems to be reasonable [63]. The application of angiotensin-converting enzyme inhibitors seems to be the only therapeutic approach that will reduce the mortality in congestive heart failure [63].

## Asymptomatic, Impaired Ventricular Ejection

If the patient is still asymptomatic but ventricular shortening is impaired (fractional shortening <25%), pharmacological afterload reduction (using captopril or enalapril) is indicated to improve ventricular ejection. If cardiac performance is not normalized by angiotensin-converting enzyme inhibitors alone, intropic support using digoxin and administration of diuretics to reduce preload should be considered. However, with the exception of angiotensin-converting enzyme inhibition to reduce afterload, it is unknown if the application of digoxin and diuretics improves the outcome or helps to postpone symptomatic heart failure [63].

## Symptomatic Heart Failure

When the patient has symptomatic heart failure, the fractional shortening is usually severely depressed (fractional shortening <15–20%), and concomitantly afterload and preload are usually increased. Treatment should include afterload reduction using captopril or enalapril, monitoring the blood pressure carefully. Additionally, inotropy should be increased using digitalis to improve the contractile state, which concomitantly will reduce afterload by reducing the end-systolic dimension. Preload should be reduced using diuretics as anticongestive therapy.

Careful monitoring for ventricular arrhythmias is mandatory, as these are a poor prognostic sign, indicating a high risk of sudden death or cardiac decompensation. In our experience the treatment of choice for ventricular arrhythmias in patients with dilative cardiomyopathy is the administration of amiodarone. Although this drug is rather toxic, it seems to be the only effective antiarrhythmic drug for these patients. As the ventricular arrhythmias are usually secondary to the cardiomyopathy, implantable defibrillators are rarely indicated.

Cardiac transplantation should be discussed early when symptomatic heart failure occurs. The timing of cardiac transplantation is still a problem, decompensated cardiomyopathy being the rule before the decision to transplant is made.

### End-Stage Cardiomyopathy

The only effective treatment for end-stage dilative cardiomyopathy and life-threatening ventricular arrhythmias is cardiac transplantation. The decision to proceed depends on the severity of clinical symptoms, a severely reduced ejection fraction, and a progressive course to the disease. However, timing of cardiac transplantation is also a problem in this particular group of patients, and decompensated cardiomyopathy is the rule here, too, before cardiac transplantation is performed.

In decompensated cardiomyopathy, aggressive pharmacological treatment, including the administration of catecholamines, enoximone, diuretics, and, in the case of ventricular tachycardias, amiodarone, is given to prevent multiorgan failure. If pharmacological treatment fails and multiorgan failure develops, the implantation of an "assist device" (an artificial heart) is the only way to keep the patient alive until cardiac transplantation becomes possible.

In conclusion, not only does the serial evaluation of cardiac function to evaluate the incidence and natural course of late anthracycline cardiotoxicity seem to be mandatory in patients treated with anthracyclines in childhood, but also the development and evaluation of therapeutic strategies for the treatment of this entity are needed to improve the outcome and quality of life for these patients.

## REFERENCES

1. Pratt CB, Ransom JL, Evans WE: Age-related Adriamycin cardiotoxicity in children. Cancer Treat Rep 62:1381–1385, 1978.
2. Goorin AM, Borow KM, Goldman A, Williams RG, Henderson IC, Sallan SE, Cohen H, Jaffe N: Congestive heart failure due to Adriamycin cardiotoxicity: Its natural history in children. Cancer 47:2810–2816, 1981.
3. Gottdiener JS, Mathisen DJ, Borer JS, Bonow RO, Myers CE, Barr LH, Schwartz DE, Bacharach SL, Green MV, Rosenberg SA: Doxorubicin cardiotoxicity: Assessment of late left ventricular dysfunction by radionuclide cineangiography. Ann Intern Med 94:430–435, 1981.
4. Lipshultz SE, Colan SD, Gelber RD, Perez-Atayde AR, Sallan SE, Sanders SP: Late cardiac effects of doxorubicin therapy for acute lymphoblastic leukemia in childhood. N Engl J Med 324:808–815, 1991.
5. Steinherz LJ, Steinherz PG, Tan CT, Heller G, Murphy ML: Cardiac toxicity 4 to 20 years after completing anthracycline therapy. J Am Med Assoc 266:1672–1677, 1991.
6. Billingham ME, Mason JW, Bristow MR, Daniels JR: Anthracycline cardiomyopathy monitored by morphologic changes. Cancer Treat Rep 62:865–872, 1978.

7. Mason JW, Bristow MR, Billingham ME, Daniel JR: Invasive and non-invasive methods of assessing Adriamycin cardiotoxic effects in man: Superiority of histopathologic assessment using endomyocardial biopsy. Cancer Treat Rep 62:857–864, 1978.

8. Ewer MS, Khalil A, Mackay B, Wallace S, Valdivieso M, Legha Ss, Benjamin RS, Haynie TP: A comparison of cardiac biopsy grades and ejection fraction estimations in patients receiving adriamycin. J Clin Oncol 2:112–117, 1984.

9. Pegelow CH, Popper RW, deWit SA, King OY, Wilbur JR: Endomyocardial biopsy to monitor anthracycline therapy in children. J Clin Oncol 2:443–446, 1984.

10. Bristow MR, Mason JW, Billingham ME, Daniels JR: Doxorubicin cardiomyopathy: Evaluation by phonocardiography, endomyocardial biopsy, and cardiac catherization. Ann Intern Med 88:168–175, 1978.

11. Braunwald E (ed): Assessment of cardiac function. In: Heart Disease. Philadelphia: W.B. Saunders, 1984, pp 409–427.

12. Glower DD, Spratt JA, Snow ND, Kabas JS, Davies JW, Olsen CO, Tyson GS, Sabiston DC, Rankin JS: Linearity of the Frank-Starling relationship in the intact heart: The concept of recruitable stroke work. Circulation 71:994–1009, 1985.

13. Ross J: Afterload mismatch and preload reserve: A conceptual framework for the analysis of ventricular function. Prog Cardiovasc Dis 18:155–164, 1976.

14. Hausdorf G, Morf G, Beron G, Erttman R, Winkler K, Landbeck G, Keck EW: Long-term doxorubicin cardiotoxicity in childhood: Noninvasive evaluation of the contractile state and diastolic filling. Br Heart J 60:309–315, 1988.

15. Bonow RD, Ostrow HG, Rosing DR, Cannon RO, Lipson LC, Maron BJ, Kent KM, Bacharach SL, Green MV: Effects of verapamil on left ventricular systolic and diastolic function in patients with hypertrophic cardiomyopathy: Pressure–volume analysis with a nonimaging scintillation probe. Circulation 68:1062–1073, 1983.

16. Devereux RB, Reichek N: Echocardiographic determinations of left ventricular mass in man. Anatomic validation of the method. Circulation 55:613–618, 1977.

17. Feigenbaum H, Popp RL, Wolfe SB, Troy BL, Pombo JF, Haine CL, Dodge HT: Ultrasound measurements of the left ventricle. Arch Intern Med 129:461–467, 1972.

18. Fortuin NJ, Hood WP, Craige E: Evaluation of left ventricular function by echocardiography. Circulation 46:26–35, 1972.

19. Lapido GOA, Dunn FG, Pringle TH, Bastian B, Lawrie TDV: Serial measurements of left ventricular dimensions by echocardiography. Br Heart J 44:1072–1083, 1980.

20. Pombo JF, Troy BL, Russel RO: Left ventricular volumes and ejection fraction by echocardiography. Circulation 43:480–490, 1971.

21. Lapido GOA, Dunn FG, Pringle TH, Bastian B, Lawrie TDV: Serial measurements of left ventricular dimensions by echocardiograpy. Br Heart J 44:1072–1083, 1980.

22. Pombo JF, Troy BL, Russel RO: Left ventricular volumes and ejection fraction by echocardiography. Circulation 43:480–490, 1971.

23. Troy BL, Pombo J, Rackley CE: Measurement of left ventricular wall thickness and mass by echocardiography. Circulation 45:602–611, 1972.

24. Sahn DJ, DeMaria A, Kissio J, Weyman A: The committee on M- mode standardization of the American Society of Echocardiography. Recommendations regarding quantification in M-mode echocardiography: Results of a survey of echocardiographic measurements. Circulation 58:1072–1083, 1978.

25. Brodie BR, McLaurin LP, Grossman W: Combined hemodynamic–ultrasonic method for studying left ventricular wall stress. Am J Cardiol 37:864–870, 1976.

26. Borow KM, Green LH, Grossman W, Braunwald E: Left ventricular end-systolic stress-shortening and stress–length relations in humans. Am J Cardiol 50:1301–1308, 1982.

27. Borow KM, Newburger JW: Non-invasive estimation of central aortic pressure using the oscillometric method for analyzing systemic artery pulsatile blood flow: Comparative study of indirect systolic, diastolic, and mean brachial artery pressure with simultaneous direct ascending aortic pressure measurements. Am Heart J 103:879–886, 1982.

28. Colan SD, Borow KM, Gamble WJ, Sanders SP: Effects of enhanced afterload (methoxamine) and contractile state (dobutamine) on the left ventricular late-systolic wall stress–dimension relation. Am J Cardiol 52:1304–1309, 1983.

29. Reichek N, Wilson J, St John Sutton M, Plappert TA, Goldberg S, Hirschfeldt JW: Non-invasive determination of left ventricular end-systolic wall stress: Validation of the method and initial application. Circulation 65:99–108, 1982.

30. Stefadouros MA, Dougherty MJ, Grossman W, Craig E: Determination of systemic vascular resistance by a non-invasive technique. Circulation 47:101–107, 1973.

31. Hausdorf G, Gluth J, Nienaber CA: Non-invasive assessment of end-systolic pressure–length and

stress-shortening relationships in normal individuals: Significance of different loading conditions induced by methoxamine and angiotensin II. Eur Heart J 8:1099–1108, 1987.

32. Laskey WK, St John Sutton M, Zeevi G, Hirschfeld JW, Reichek N: Left ventricular mechanics in dilated cardiomyopathy. Am J Cardiol 54:620–625, 1984.

33. Chen W, Gibson DG: Relation of isovolumic relaxation to left ventricular wall motion in man. Br Heart J 45:122–128, 1981.

34. Gibson DG, Brown D: Measurement of instantaneous left ventricular dimension and filling rate in man using echocardiography. Br Heart J 35:1141–1149, 1973.

35. Hanrath P, Mathey DG, Siegert R, Bleifeld W: Left ventricular relaxation and filling pattern in different forms of left ventricular hypertrophy. Am J Cardiol 45:15–23, 1980.

36. Upton MT, Gibson DG: The study of left ventricular function from digitized echocardiograms. Prog Cardiovasc Dis 20:359–384, 1978.

37. Zoghbi WA, Habib GB, Quinones MA: Doppler assessment of right ventricular filling in a normal population. Comparison with left ventricular filling dynamics. Circulation 82:1316–1324, 1990.

38. DeMaria AN, Wisenbaugh TW, Smith MD, Harrison MR, Berk MR: Doppler echocardiography evaluation of diastolic dysfunction. Circulation 84(suppl 1):I-288–I-295, 1991.

39. Voutilainen S, Kupari M, Hippelainen M, Karpinnen K, Ventila M, Heikkila J: Factors influencing Doppler indexes of left ventricular filling in healthy persons. Am J Cardiol 68:653–659, 1991.

40. Goldberg SJ, Hutter JJ, Feldman L, Goldberg SM: Two sensitive echocardiographic techniques for detecting doxorubicin toxicity. Med Pediatr Oncol 11:172–177, 1983.

41. Gibson DG, Brown DJ: Continuous assessment of left ventricular shape in man. Br Heart J 37:904–910, 1975.

42. Gould KL, Lipscomb K, Hamilton GW, Kennedy JW: Relation of left ventricular shape, function, and wall stress in man. Am J Cardiol 34:627–634, 1974.

43. Lange PE, Onnasch D, Farr FL, Heintzen PH: Angiocardiographic left ventricular volume determination. Accuracy, as determined from human casts and clinical applications. Eur J Cardiol 8:449–476, 1978.

44. Weber KT, Kinasewitz GT, Janicki JS, Fishman AP: Oxygen utilization and ventilation during exercise in patients with chronic cardiac failure. Circulation 65:1213–1223, 1982.

45. Webert KT, Kanicki JS, McElroy PA: Determination of aerobic capacity and the severity of chronic cardiac and circulatory failure. Circulation 79(suppl 6):VI-40–VI-45, 1978.

46. Bristow JD, Kloster FE, Lees MH, Menashe VD, Grisworld HE, Starr A: Serial cardiac catheterizations and exercise hemodynamics after correction of tetralogy of Fallot. Circulation 41:1057–1066, 1970.

47. Wessel HU, Cunningham WJ, Paul MH, Bastanier CK, Muster AJ, Idriss FS: Exercise performance in tetralogy of Fallot after intracardiac repair. J Thorac Cardiovasc Surg 80:582–593, 1980.

48. Slutsky R: Response of the left ventricle to stress: Effects of exercise, atrial pacing, afterload stress and drugs. Am J Cardiol 47:357–364, 1981.

49. Borow KM, Propper R, Bierman FZ, Grady S, Inati A: The left ventricular end-systolic pressure–dimension relation in patients with thalassemia major. Circulation 66:980–985, 1982.

50. Borow KM, Neumann A, Wynne J: Sensitivity of end-systolic pressure–dimension and pressure–volume relations to the inotropic state in humans. Circulation 65:988–997, 1982.

51. Borow KM, Henderson C, Neumann A, Colan S, Grady S, Papish S, Goorin A: Assessment of left ventricular contractility in patients receiving doxorubicin. Ann Intern Med 99:750–756, 1983.

52. Kono A, Maughan L, Sunagawa K, Hamilton K, Sagawa K, Weisfeldt ML: The use of left ventricular end-ejection pressure and peak pressure in the estimation of the end-systolic pressure–volume relationship. Circulation 70:1057–1065, 1984.

53. Mehmel HC, Stockins B, Ruffman K, Ohlshausen K, Schuler G, Kuebler W: The linearity of the end-systolic pressure–volume relationship in man and its sensitivity for the assessment of left ventricular function. Circulation 63:1216–1222, 1981.

54. Sagawa K: Editorial: The end-systolic pressure–volume relation of the ventricle: Definition, modifications and clinical use. Circulation 63:1223–1227, 1981.

55. Weber KT, Janicki JS, Hunter WC, Shroff S, Pearlman ES, Fishman AP: The contractile behaviour of the heart and its functional coupling to the circulation. Prog Cardiovasc Dis 24:375–400, 1982.

56. Lang RM, Borow KM, Neumann A, Janzen D: Systemic vascular resistance: An unreliable index of left ventricular afterload. Circulation 74:1114–1123, 1986.

57. Colan SD, Borow KM, Neumann A: Left ventricular end-systolic wall stress velocity of fiber

shortening relation: A load independent index of myocardial contractility. J Am Coll Cardiol 4:715–724, 1984.

58. Hausdorf G, Rettig TH, Keck EW: Evaluation of left ventricular contractile performance from baseline stress-shortening data in man: Comparison with pharmacological afterload challenge. Clin Cardiol 11:764–770, 1988.

59. Mortensen SA, Olsen HS, Baandrup U: Chronic anthracycline cardiotoxicity: Hemodynamic and histopathological manifestations suggesting a restrictive endomyocardial disease. Br Heart J 55:274–282, 1986.

60. Mirsky I: Assessment of passive diastolic stiffness of cardiac muscle: Mathematical concepts, physiologic and clinical considerations, directions of future research. Prog Cardiovasc Dis 18:277–308, 1976.

61. Hess OM, Grimm J, Krayenbuehl HP: Diastolic simple elastic and viscoelastic properties of the human left ventricle in man. Circulation 59:1178–1187, 1979.

62. Hess OM, Schneider J, Koch R, Bamert C, Grimm J, Krayenbuehl HP: Diastolic function and myocardial structure in patients with myocardial hypertrophy. Special reference to normalized viscoelastic data. Circulation 63:360–371, 1981.

63. The CONSENSUS Trial Group. Effect of enalapril on mortality in severe congestive heart failure. N Engl J Med 316:1429–1435, 1987.

# 9. Cardiac Function Following Cardiotoxic Therapy During Childhood: Assessing the Damage

Regina I. Jakacki, M.D., Ranae L. Larsen, M.D., Gerald Barber, M.D., Joel W. Goldwein, M.D., and Jeffrey H. Silber, M.D., Ph.D.

The cardiotoxicity of both the anthracyclines and heart irradiation has been apparent since the 1960s [1,2] but remains poorly understood and continues to be their dose-limiting toxicity. Both modalities may have long-term effects on the heart [3,4], and the added impact of aging and atherosclerosis compound the potential for late sequelae. More and more reports are surfacing of unexpected sudden deaths and onset of congestive heart failure long after therapy has been discontinued [5,6]. Because there is a long life expectancy following successful treatment of childhood cancer, it is important to identify those patients who have sustained significant damage to their hearts and are therefore at risk for further problems.

We used a battery of noninvasive tests to evaluate cardiac function in 205 children and young adults who had received cardiotoxic therapy for a childhood malignancy in order to: (1) define the characteristics and incidence of cardiac abnormalities in this patient population, (2) correlate the results of the studies in this battery, and (3) develop a practical algorithm for monitoring the increasing numbers of patients at risk for future cardiac problems.

## METHODS

From September 1989 to February 1991, patients whose therapy for a childhood malignancy included an anthracycline and/or irradiation that included a portion of the left ventricle in the radiation field were approached at the time of routine clinic visits to the Children's Hospital of Philadelphia Oncology Clinic and asked to participate in the study.

Each patient underwent at least three of the following tests:

1. 2-D and 2-D-directed M-mode echocardiogram for determination of shortening fraction (SF);
2. Resting and exercise ECG-gated nuclear cardiac blood pool scans (multigated acquisition: MUGA) [7]. MUGA scans were obtained using the following protocol: After in vitro labeling of the patient's red blood cells with technetium 99m, images were obtained in a left anterior oblique position using an Anger camera and a high-sensitivity parallel-hole collimator. Resting left ventricular ejection fractions (LVEF) were determined and Fourier analysis for regional wall motion abnormality was performed while the patient was supine and again in the semierect

position. Symptom-limited exercise testing was performed in the semierect position, with images obtained at graded workloads that were increased at 3-minute intervals.

3. Resting electrocardiogram (ECG);

4. 24-hour Holter monitor;

5. A questionnaire regarding exercise ability and history of symptoms with exercise. Response to the following question was evaluated: Do you/Does your child complain of difficulty during or following physical exertion?

6. Cardiopulmonary exercise testing using cycle ergometry. Cardiac output was measured by an acetylene–helium–carbon monoxide rebreathing technique [8] at rest and every 3 minutes throughout exercise and was indexed for body surface area. All patients were encouraged to exercise to the point of exhaustion.

The cardiopulmonary exercise test and resting and exercise cardiac scan were done on separate days (median interval between tests: 1 month). For patients off therapy, all tests were done within 6 months of each other. For those patients who were still receiving chemotherapy, the testing was not done within 3 weeks of the last dose of anthracycline and all tests were performed prior to the subsequent dose. No patient had evidence of congestive heart failure at the time of study.

Table 1 shows the battery of tests and the parameters used to define a study as abnormal.

## RESULTS

### Abnormalities in Anthracycline-Treated Patients

Table 2 shows the frequency of abnormalities in 140 patients who had received at least one dose of anthracycline (ANTH) and were at least 3 months from their last dose. There was an increase in abnormalities detected on the resting MUGA, but no

**TABLE 1. Cardiac Function Testing**

| Test | Definition of Abnormal |
|---|---|
| Echocardiogram | Shortening Fraction (SF) <28% [10] |
| Resting MUGA | Supine ejection fraction (EF) <55% |
| | Presence of or abnormal wall motion |
| Exercise MUGA | Fall in ejection fraction below resting semierect value |
| Cardiopulmonary exercise test | Maximal cardiac index (MCI) >2 SD below normal laboratory values |
| Electrocardiogram (ECG) | $QT_c$ interval > 0.44 [11] |
| 24-hour Holter monitor | Presence of supraventricular or ventricular tachycardia or ventricular couplet |

**TABLE 2. Cardiac Function Abnormalities in Patients More Than 3 Months From Last Anthracycline**

| N = 146 | |
|---|---|
| Age:[a] | 15.4 yr (7.2–28.9 yr) |
| Age at treatment: | 9.1 yr (2.8 mo–19.3 yr) |
| Time from last ANTH dose: | 5.1 yr (3.2 mo–17.2 yr) |
| ANTH dose: | 311 mg/$M^2$ (84–750) |
| Number receiving radiation: | 46 |

| Test | No. Abnormal/Total (%) |
|---|---|
| Echocardiogram SF <28% | 11/131 (8.4%) |
| Radionuclide scan (MUGA) Resting EF <55% | 21/72 (29.2%) |
| Electrocardiogram $QT_c$ > 0.44 | 22/145 (15.2%) |
| 24-hour Holter monitor significant dysrhythmia | 8/121 (6.6%) |
| Cardiopulmonary exercise test MCI <5th %ile | 64/146 (43.8%) |

[a]Mean, (range).

SF, shortening fraction; EF, ejection fraction; MCI, maximal cardiac index.

other test, as time from last ANTH dose increased. Twelve of 27 (44.4%) patients at least 5 years from their last ANTH dose had a resting ejection fraction (EF) <55% versus 9/45 (20%) patients between 3 months and 5 years from completion of ANTH. However, after adjusting for dose and age at treatment, the effect of follow-up time was of borderline significance ($P$ = .06).

## Abnormalities in "Low-Risk" Patients

Table 3 shows the frequency of abnormalities seen in a subgroup of 64 patients who would traditionally be considered

**TABLE 3. Cardiac Function Abnormalities in "Low-Risk" Patients More Than 3 Months From Anthracycline or Irradiation**

|  | N = 64 |
|---|---|
| Sex: | 30 females, 34 males |
| Age:[a] | 16.3 yr (8.2–28.9) |
| Time from cardiac therapy: | 5.6 yr (3.2 mo–17.2 yr) |
| Age at treatment: | 9.8 yr (6.6 mo–19.3 yr) |
| ANTH dose (N = 61): | 248 mg/M² (84–347) |
| Radiation dose to left ventricle (N = 3): | 613 cGy (480–760) |

| Test | No. Abnormal/Total (%) |
|---|---|
| Echocardiogram | |
| SF <28% | 4/56 (7.1%) |
| Radionuclide scan (MUGA) | |
| Resting EF <55% | 5/29 (17.2%) |
| Fall in EF with exercise | 4/29 (13.8%) |
| Both resting and exercise abnormal | 1/29 (3.4%) |
| Electrocardiogram | |
| QT$_c$ > 0.44 | 2/64 (3.1%) |
| 24-hour Holter monitor significant dysrhythmia (SVT) | 1/53 (1.9%) |
| Cardiopulmonary exercise test | |
| MCI <5th %ile | 20/63 (31.7%) |

[a]Mean (range)
SF, shortening fraction; EF, ejection fraction; MCI, maximal cardiac index.

"low risk." No patient received more than 350 mg/m² of ANTH or more than a radiation index of 1,000 cGy-percent to the left ventricle (defined as the dose to the midpoint of the left ventricle multiplied by the percentage of the left ventricle in the radiation field). Patients who received spinal irradiation or both anthracycline and cardiac irradiation were excluded. Abnormalities were present in all areas of testing.

## Holter Monitoring

Twenty-four-hour Holter monitoring demonstrated conduction and rhythm abnormalities at frequencies greater than would be expected for an age-matched healthy population [12–15]. Table 4 lists the frequency of abnormalities we previously described [16] in 134 patients who were at least 3 months from completion of either ANTH or cardiac irradiation. Although most patients had abnormalities limited to single supraventricular or ventricular premature complexes, potentially serious ventricular ectopy was seen in several patients. Patients who received both anthracyclines and cardiac irradiation appeared to be at greatest risk for ventricular

**TABLE 4. Holter Abnormalities**

| (N = 134) | | |
|---|---|---|
|  | Patients[a] | Normal Children |
| Supraventricular premature complexes | (89) 66.4 | 30 |
| Supraventricular tachycardia | (3) 2.2 | 0.3 |
| Ventricular premature complexes | (70) 52.2 | 31 |
| Ventricular couplets | (5) 3.7 | 1.5 |
| Ventricular tachycardia | (4) 3 | 1.7 |
| 2nd degree AV block type II | (5) 3.7 | 0.3 |

[a](Number abnormal)/%abnormal.
[b]%Abnormal.

arrhythmias. Of the 37 patients who had received both anthracycline and left ventricular irradiation, three patients had ventricular couplets (8%) and three patients had recorded episodes of nonsustained ventricular tachycardia (8%). Anthracycline doses in the patients with ventricular tachycardia ranged from 210–300 mg/m². One additional patient with ventricular tachycardia had received cardiac irradiation alone. All of these episodes occurred while the patients were awake and no symptoms were recorded. All four patients with ventricular tachycardia had normal shortening fractions (31%–36%) and normal QT$_c$ intervals on resting ECG.

## Comparison of Tests

Seventy-three patients, 29 females and 44 males, who had received at least one dose of anthracycline underwent the entire battery of tests, and the associations between tests were examined. Primary diagnoses included acute leukemia (23 patients), non-Hodgkin's lymphoma (18 patients), Hodgkin's disease (8 patients), Wilms' tumor (9 patients), and sarcoma (15 patients). The median patient age at the time of the study was 15.3 years (range 9–28.9 years). The total anthracycline dose (doxorubicin and/or daunorubicin) ranged from 50–750 mg/m² with a median of 300 mg/m². The median time from last anthracycline was 2.7 years (range 4 weeks to 15.2 years) and the median age at the time of treatment was 9.9 years, range 8.7 months to 19.3 years. Twenty-three patients had also received therapeutic mediastinal or flank irradiation that included a portion of the heart in the radiation field (mean tumor dose 1,985 cGy, range 600 to 5,400 cGy). All patients were at least 1 month from their last dose of anthracycline. There was no difference in the frequency of abnormalities between those patients who were greater than 3 months from

their last ANTH dose and those less than 3 months, and the results were combined and are shown in Table 5.

Patients who had an abnormal shortening fraction on echocardiogram (ESF) or prolongation of the QT$_c$ interval on ECG were significantly more likely to have an abnormal resting ejection fraction on MUGA. As can be seen in Figure 1, 5/7 patients with an abnormal ESF and 7/11 patients (63.6%) with a prolonged QT$_c$ interval on ECG had an abnormal resting ejection fraction.

There was no association between abnormalities at rest and abnormalities with exercise. Six of the seven patients with an abnormal ESF had a normal ejection fraction response with exercise. Figure 2 shows the relationship between the resting MUGA and the exercise tests. Patients with an abnormal resting study were no more likely to have an abnormal exercise study than those who were normal at rest. A history of difficulty with exercise correlated better with an abnormal resting MUGA than either exercise study.

**TABLE 5. Frequency of Abnormalities in 73 Patients Undergoing Entire Battery of Tests**

| Test | Number Abnormal | % |
|---|---|---|
| Echocardiogram | | |
| Shortening fraction | 7 | (9.6) |
| MUGA | | |
| Resting ejection fraction | 22 | (30.1) |
| EF response to exercise | 9 | (12.3) |
| Both resting and exercise | 4 | (5.0) |
| Electrocardiogram | | |
| QT$_c$ prolongation | 11 | (15.1) |
| 24-hour Holter monitor | | |
| Significant dysrhythmia | 6 | (8.2) |
| Questionnaire | | |
| Complaints of "difficulty" during or after physical exertion | 35 | (47.9) |
| Cardiopulmonary exercise test (N = 68 evaluable) | 26 | (38.2) |

## RESTING MUGA ASSOCIATIONS

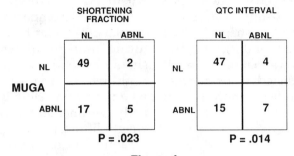

Figure 1.

## RESTING MUGA / EXERCISE ASSESSMENT ASSOCIATIONS

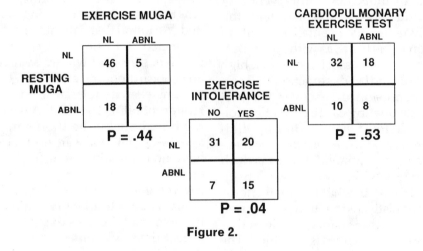

Figure 2.

There was no association between the two exercise tests. Indeed, five of seven patients (71%) who had a fall in ejection fraction with exercise on MUGA were able to achieve a normal maximal cardiac index on cycle ergometry.

### Algorithm for Screening

The MUGA is considered by many to be the most reliable noninvasive means of detecting subclinical left ventricular dysfunction and is generally considered the method of choice for monitoring anthracycline use in adults [17–19]. However, it is expensive, entails a small biologic hazard, and is not always practical for general use. We examined the tests that had a strong association with an abnormal resting ejection fraction on MUGA (QT$_c$ interval on ECG, shortening fraction on echocardiography, and complaints of difficulty with exercise on questionnaire), in order to identify patients for whom a MUGA may not be necessary.

The algorithm would predict that patients with a normal ESF and $QT_c$ interval and no complaints of exercise intolerance would have a normal resting MUGA. Using this algorithm, 29 of 73 patients (39.7%) would have avoided undergoing the MUGA. Figure 3 shows that only 2 of 29 patients (6.9%) predicted to be normal would actually have been abnormal on testing.

## DISCUSSION

It is becoming increasingly apparent that even what were previously considered "safe" doses of anthracycline carry a risk of cardiac damage. All patients whose treatment included an anthracycline or cardiac irradiation deserve long-term follow-up. Even relatively small amounts of irradiation to the heart, as with spinal irradiation, have been associated with a high incidence of cardiac dysfunction [20].

Much confusion exists over the best means of evaluating cardiac function following cardiotoxic therapy during childhood. There are many methods for screening and many recommendations on which method to use, while there is also considerable variability in what is actually done. As more sophisticated techniques are coming into use, the chance of detecting subclinical abnormalities is very high. The

significance of many of these findings and whether they predict for subsequent clinical cardiac decompensation is not known. Until these are clarified, the goals of monitoring (outside of research protocols) should be to identify those patients who could benefit from early intervention or who need counseling in regard to potentially detrimental lifestyle practices (e.g., weight lifting, smoking, alcohol, etc.).

Monitoring of the ever-increasing population of survivors of childhood cancer is often less than optimal because of practical constraints of time, money, and availability of technical resources. Many of these children are followed as young adults by physicians in the community where access to more advanced testing may be limited. We found that patients could be safely "screened" by using four relatively inexpensive, safe, and widely available tests: an echocardiogram, an ECG, a history regarding exercise tolerance, and a 24-hour Holter monitor. The MUGA was unlikely to be abnormal if the shortening fraction and the $QT_c$ interval were normal and there were no complaints of difficulty with exercise.

Twelve-lead electrocardiography alone is inadequate to identify patients at risk for potentially serious dysrhythmias, and in fact there was no association between dysrhythmias on Holter monitoring and studies of resting cardiac function. Prolongation of the $QT_c$ interval is associated with myocardial instability and is seen in syndromes with a high incidence of dysrhythmias and sudden death [21]. However, none of the patients with ventricular tachycardia and only one of the five patients with ventricular couplets had a prolonged $QT_c$ interval on ECG. Ventricular ectopy that may be benign in patients without underlying heart disease is more serious in patients with cardiomyopathies [22]. There have been no prospective studies on the significance of ven-

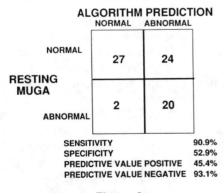

ALGORITHM PREDICTION

|  | NORMAL | ABNORMAL |
|---|---|---|
| **NORMAL** | 27 | 24 |
| **ABNORMAL** | 2 | 20 |

RESTING MUGA

| | |
|---|---|
| SENSITIVITY | 90.9% |
| SPECIFICITY | 52.9% |
| PREDICTIVE VALUE POSITIVE | 45.4% |
| PREDICTIVE VALUE NEGATIVE | 93.1% |

Figure 3.

tricular ectopy in patients who have received cardiotoxic therapy for malignancies. Steinherz et al., however, reported arrhythmias as the cause of death in two patients who died suddenly years after cardiotoxic therapy was discontinued [23]. Unlike their patients, none of our patients with ventricular tachycardia had evidence of systolic dysfunction on echocardiography and no patient had received more than 300 mg/m² of anthracycline.

The exact pathophysiology of anthracycline-induced cardiomyopathy is unclear. One theory as to why the pathologic myocardial damage can remain asymptomatic for so long is that physiologic reserve and compensatory responses are able to maintain normal cardiac function until a certain threshold is reached, reflecting both reversible and irreversible structural damage [24]. The first manifestations of cardiac dysfunction are often symptoms with exercise. As a consequence, exercise testing has been used as a means of uncovering abnormalities not detectable at rest. It was therefore somewhat surprising to find that there was no association between abnormalities at rest and abnormalities with exercise, and that many of those with an abnormal resting study were able to achieve a normal exercise response. Since not all normal children increase their ejection fraction wtih exercise [25], an isolated abnormality on exercise testing is of unclear clinical significance.

In summary, patients who have received anthracyclines or radiation to the heart should have long-term cardiac follow-up, regardless of dose. Those patients with a normal echocardiogram, $QT_c$ interval on ECG, and no history of exercise intolerance are unlikely to have an abnormal MUGA. Significant dysrhythmias may be present in the absence of other abnormalities, particularly in patients who received both anthracyclines and cardiac irradiation.

# REFERENCES

1. Stewart JR, Cohn KE, Fajardo LF, Hancock EW, Kaplan HS: Radiation induced heart disease. Radiology 89:302–310, 1967.
2. Bonadonna G, Monfardini S: Cardiac toxicity of daunorubicin. Lancet 1:837, 1969.
3. Gottdiener JS, Katin MJ, Borer JS, Bacharach SL, Green MV: Late cardiac effects of therapeutic mediastinal irradiation: Assessment by echocardiography and radionuclide angiography. N Engl J Med 308:569–572, 1983.
4. Von Hoff DD, Rozencweig M, Layard M, et al.: Daunomycin-induced cardiotoxicity in children and adults. Am J Med 62:200–208, 1977.
5. Goorin AM, Chauvenet AR, Perez-Atayde AR, Perez-Atayde AR, Sallan SA, Sauders SP: Initial congestive heart failure six to ten years after doxorubicin chemotherapy for childhood cancer. J Pediatr 116:144–147, 1990.
6. Hawkins MM, Kingston JE, Kinnier Wilson LM: Late deaths after treatment for childhood cancer. Arch Dis Child 65:1356–1363, 1990.
7. Green MV, Ostrow MG, Douglas MA, et al.: High temporal resolution ECG gated scintigraphic angiocardiography. J Nucl Med 16:95–98, 1975.
8. Triebwasser JH, Johnson RL, Burpo RP, et al.: Noninvasive determination of cardiac output by a modified acetylene rebreathing procedure utilizing mass spectrometer measurements. Aviation Space Environ Med 48:203–209, 1977.
9. Zavala DC: Manual on exercise testing: A training handbook. Iowa City, IA: University of Iowa Press, 1987, p 51.
10. Feigenbaum H: Echocardiography, 4th ed. Philadelphia: Lea and Febiger, 1986, pp 621–624.
11. Park MK, Gunteroth WG: How to Read Pediatric ECGs. Chicago: Yearbook Medical Publishers, 1987, pp 217–218.
12. Scott O, Williams GJ, Fiddler GI: Results of 24 hour ambulatory monitoring of electrocardiogram in 131 healthy boys aged 10–13 years. Br Heart J 44:304–308, 1980.
13. Southall DP, Johnston F, Shinebourne EA, Johnston PGB: 24-hour electrocardiographic study of heart rate and rhythm patterns in a population of healthy children. Br Heart J 45:281–291, 1981.
14. Brodsky M, Wu D, Denes P, Kanakis C, Rosen KM: Arrhythmias documented by 24-hour continuous electrocardiographic monitoring in 50 male medical students without apparent heart disease. Am J Card 39:390–395, 1977.

15. Dickinson DF, Scott O: Ambulatory electrocardiographic monitoring in 100 healthy teenage boys. Br Heart J 51:179–183, 1984.
16. Larsen RL, Jakacki RI, Vetter VL, Meadows AT, Silber JH, Barber G: Electrocardiographic changes and arrhythmias after cancer therapy in children and young adults. Am J Cardiol 70:73–77, 1992.
17. Druck MN, Gulenchy KY, Evans WK, et al.: Radionuclide angiography and endomyocardial biopsy in the assessment of doxorubicin cardiotoxicity. Cancer 53:1667–1674, 1984.
18. Alexander J, Dainiak N, Berger HJ, et al.: Serial assessment of doxorubicin cardiotoxicity with quantitative radionuclide angiocardiography. N Engl J Med 300:278–283, 1979.
19. Schwartz RG, McKenzie WB, Alexander J, et al.: Congestive heart failure and left ventricular dysfunction complicating doxorubicin therapy. Am J Med 82:1109–1118, 1987.
20. Jakacki RI, Larsen R, Goldwein J, Silber J, et al.: Cardiotoxicity of spinal irradiation in pediatric central nervous system tumors. Proc Am Soc Clin Oncol 10:365, 1991 (abstr).
21. Schwartz PJ, Periti M, Malliani A: The long Q-T syndrome. Am Heart J 89:378, 1975.
22. Maron BJ, Savage DD, Wolfson JK, Epstein SE: Prognostic significance of 24 hour ambulatory electrocardiographic monitoring in patients with hypertrophic cardiomyopathy: A prospective study. Am J Cardiol 48:252–257, 1981.
23. Steinherz LJ, Steinherz PG, Tan CT, Heller G, Murphy L: Cardiac toxicity 4 to 20 years after completing anthracycline therapy. J Am Med Assoc 266:1672–1677, 1991.
24. Young RD, Ozols RF, Myers CE: The anthracycline antineoplastic drugs. N Engl J Med 305(3):139–153, 1981.
25. Parrish MD, Boucek RJ, Burger J, et al.: Exercise radionuclide ventriculography in children: Normal values for exercise variables and right and left ventricular function. Br Heart J 54:509–516, 1985.

# 10. Forecasting Cardiac Function After Anthracyclines in Childhood: The Role of Dose, Age, and Gender

Jeffrey H. Silber, M.D.,Ph.D., Regina I. Jakacki, M.D.,
Ranae L. Larsen, M.D., Joel W. Goldwein, M.D., and Gerald Barber, M.D.

In the 1970s, anthracyclines were associated with major advances in the treatment of many tumors. Balanced against this success was the belief that about 5% of patients treated with cumulative doses (of doxorubicin) near 540 mg/m² would develop congestive heart failure, and that most of these episodes would be fatal [1–3]. The benefits of these drugs seemed to outweigh their risks, and consequently the use of anthracyclines increased. However, recent reports have shown a wide range of cardiac abnormalities other than congestive heart failure that may follow anthracycline administration during childhood [4–6].

Today, we are faced with a very different portfolio of uses for anthracyclines, in part because of the many early successes. Anthracyclines are now used as first-line therapy in many common malignancies, including childhood leukemias [7] and the treatment of early-stage Hodgkin's disease [8]. As the applications for anthracyclines increase, benefits from treatment may, at times, become more marginal [9]. In the case of early-stage Hodgkin's disease, for example, the addition of anthracyclines is motivated more by a desire to avoid side effects from alkylating agents than the expectation of better survival rates. When substitutes for anthracyclines are available, the relative importance of the cardiac risks of anthracyclines greatly increases. Consequently, the development of frank congestive heart failure may not be the only relevant outcome measure by which to evaluate anthracycline cardiotoxicity. Patients and their families are concerned about any clinically abnormal cardiac function (not only the avoidance of a potentially lethal side effect such as congestive heart failure). We therefore sought to develop a model that would predict abnormalities with exercise or at rest and thus to better quantify the risks of anthracycline cardiac dysfunction. Such a model would help guide clinicians when only marginal benefits from anthracyclines are expected or when substitutes for anthracyclines may be available, as in the Hodgkin's disease example cited.

The analysis was based on the cumulative dose of anthracycline, age, and gender. Our intent was to use an outcome measure sensitive enough to identify abnormalities possibly not apparent at rest. Therefore exercise testing was included.

## METHODS

### Patient Selection

Patients were eligible to enroll in this study if they met the following criteria. All patients must have been: (1) followed by the Pediatric Oncology Clinic at the Children's Hospital of Philadelphia; (2) treated for cancer with anthracyclines, with or without heart irradiation (and excluding spinal axis irradiation); (3) tall enough to reach the bicycle pedals for exercise testing (a minimum of 115 cm); and (4) at least 1 month beyond their last dose of anthracycline. Informed consent was obtained from all patients or their guardians, and the study was approved by our institutional review board.

In order to better delineate the cardiac effects of cancer therapy, from September 1989 to February 1991 exercise testing was performed on 205 patients from the Children's Hospital of Philadelphia Oncology Clinic. We excluded 37 patients who did not receive anthracyclines; nine patients who received spinal axis irradiation (a risk factor for cardiotoxicity [10]); and eight patients who were less than 1 month beyond anthracycline administration or heart irradiation. This left 151 patients available for analysis.

## Cardiac Evaluation

Each patient received one or both of the following tests: (1) resting and exercise nuclear cardiac blood pool scans (MUGA), using the standard electrocardiogram (ECG) gating techniques [11–13]. The technique was as follows: After *in vitro* labeling of the patient's red blood cells with technetium 99m, images were obtained in a left anterior oblique position using an Anger camera and a high-sensitivity parallel-hole collimator. Resting left ventricular ejection fractions (LVEF) were determined and Fourier analysis for regional wall-motion abnormality was performed while the patient was supine and again in the semierect position. Exercise testing was performed in the semierect position, with images obtained at graded workloads that were increased at 3-minute intervals. An abnormal resting supine ejection fraction was defined as <55% or the presence of abnormal wall motion. An abnormal exercise MUGA was defined as a maximal ejection fraction less than the resting semierect value.

(2) Exercise testing was performed using standard cycle ergometry with ECG monitoring [14,15]. Cardiac output measured by an acetylene–helium–carbon monoxide rebreathing technique [16,17] at rest and every 3 minutes throughout exercise was indexed to body surface area. All patients were encouraged to exercise to the point of exhaustion. Abnormal results were defined as greater than 1.64 standard deviations (SD) below normal values ( 7.1 L/min/m$^2$) determined in our cardiopulmonary exercise laboratory on 60 normal subjects, correcting for body surface area at the time of the cardiac study.

## Statistical Methods

Multiple logistic regression was used to predict the probability of having an abnormal response on either or both tests. The adjusted relative risk was computed from the calculated odds ratio, with the associated 95% confidence interval. Total anthracycline dose was defined as total dose of doxorubicin plus total dose of daunorubicin in mg/m$^2$.

## RESULTS

The distribution of primary diagnoses was as follows: acute lymphoblastic leukemia, 20 patients; acute nonlymphoblastic leukemia, 23 patients; non-Hodgkin's lymphoma, 27 patients; Hodgkin's disease, 21 patients; sarcomas, 29 patients; Wilms' tumor, 23 patients; and other rarer malignancies, 8 patients.

A further description of the patient population is displayed in Table 1. Most patients received anthracyclines without

**TABLE 1.  Patient Description**

| | |
|---|---|
| Number of patients | 151 |
| Gender (M:F) | 85:66 |
| Age when treated (years) | |
|    Mean ± SD | 9.5 ± 5.1 |
|    Range (min, max) | (0.23, 21) |
| Age when studied (years) | |
|    Mean ± SD | 15.5 ± 4.5 |
|    Range (min, max) | (7, 29) |
| Years between treatment and study | |
|    Mean ± SD | 4.7 ± 4.0 |
|    Range (min, max) | (0.09, 18) |
| Total anthracycline dose | |
|    Mean ± SD | 307 ± 120 |
|    Range (min, max) | (50, 750) |
| Number with radiation to heart | 40 |
| Total radiation dose to heart in | |
|    Gy (N = 40) | |
|    Mean ± SD | 19.6 ± 8.65 |
|    Range (min, max) | (8, 45) |
| MUGA (abnormal:normal) | 28:47 |
| Cardiac output (abnormal:normal) | 62:89 |
| MUGA or cardiac output | |
|    (one or both abnormal:both normal) | 77:74 |

irradiation; however, 40 patients received both anthracyclines and irradiation of the heart.

Variables reflecting heart irradiation were not statistically significant after accounting for gender, age, and anthracycline dose. Time from treatment also failed to reach statistical significance when added to the above model. Interactions were explored between model variables but also did not reach statistical significance.

The relationship between dose of anthracycline, age at treatment, and gender is described in Table 2, where the results of the multiple logistic regression models are displayed. The probability of developing an abnormal test increases with increasing cumulative dosage of anthracycline, younger age at time of treatment, and female gender. Note that we defined total dose of anthracycline as the total doxorubicin dose plus the total daunorubicin dose. When we compared our results to models weighing daunorubicin as less toxic than doxorubicin (i.e., using two-thirds the dose of daunorubicin plus the full dose of doxorubicin when calculating total dose), we found the latter models to be slightly inferior. Consequently, we defined total dose of anthracyclines as simply the sum of total doxorubicin plus daunorubicin in mg/m$^2$.

From the model shown in Table 2, one can compute the probability of developing an abnormal exercise test based on a patient's cumulative dose of anthracycline, age, and gender. These probabilities are displayed in Table 3 (for males and females) along with their 95% confidence intervals. The model shown in Table 2 was also used to graph the point estimates for specific doses of anthracycline received during ages 2 through 18 years. Figure 1 displays these probability estimates for males, and Figure 2 for females. Note that

**TABLE 2.  Multiple Logistic Regression Model to Predict Test Abnormality**

| Variable | Parameter Estimate | Standard Error | P Value |
|---|---|---|---|
| Anthracycline dose (mg/m$^2$) | 0.005 | 0.002 | 0.001 |
| Age at treatment (yrs) | -0.072 | 0.036 | 0.040 |
| Gender (1 = female, 0 = male) | 1.204 | 0.364 | 0.001 |
| Intercept | -1.538 | | |

Model Chi$^2$ statistic, P value = 0.0001.
C statistic = 0.73.

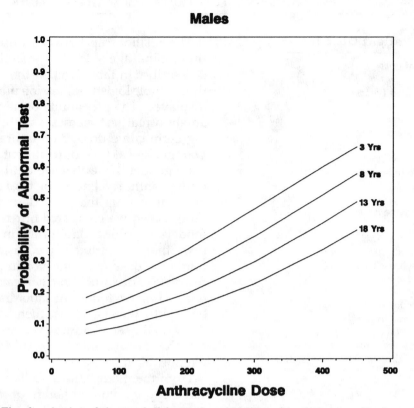

**Fig. 1.** A plot of the model-derived probability of test abnormality in males for a specified dose of anthracycline and age at treatment.

**TABLE 3.** Point Estimates and 95% Confidence Intervals for the Probability of Test Abnormality in Males and Females for a Given Age and Anthracycline Dose

| Age (yr) | 100 mg/m² | 200 mg/m² | 300 mg/m² | 400 mg/m² |
|---|---|---|---|---|
| *Males* | | | | |
| 3 | 0.229 | 0.338 | 0.467 | 0.601 |
| | (.103,.434) | (.197,.515) | (.317,.623) | (.429,.751) |
| 8 | 0.171 | 0.262 | 0.379 | 0.512 |
| | (.081,.326) | (.162,.394) | (.274,.496) | (.375,.647) |
| 13 | 0.126 | 0.198 | 0.298 | 0.422 |
| | (.055,.261) | (.113,.325) | (.197,.424) | (.282,.576) |
| 18 | 0.091 | 0.147 | 0.228 | 0.337 |
| | (.033,.225) | (.067,.293) | (.118,.394) | (.180,.541) |
| *Females* | | | | |
| 3 | 0.498 | 0.630 | 0.745 | 0.834 |
| | (.273,.723) | (.435,.790) | (.584,.859) | (.690,.919) |
| 8 | 0.408 | 0.542 | 0.670 | 0.777 |
| | (.229,.615) | (.387,.689) | (.540,.778) | (.645,.870) |
| 13 | 0.324 | 0.452 | 0.586 | 0.709 |
| | (.170,.530) | (.303,.610) | (.447,.713) | (.556,.825) |
| 18 | 0.250 | 0.365 | 0.496 | 0.629 |
| | (.110,.475) | (.202,.566) | (.316,.678) | (.423,.796) |

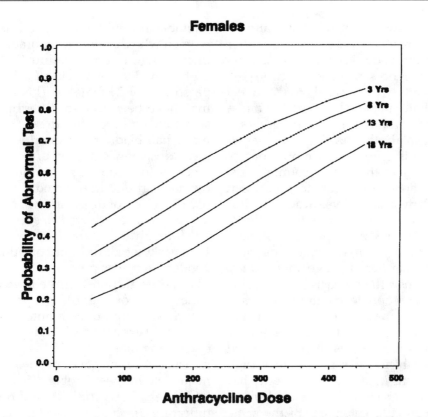

**Fig. 2.** A plot of the model-derived probability of test abnormality in females for a specified dose of anthracycline and age at treatment.

there is a considerable difference in the risk of exercise test abnormalities between high and low doses of anthracyclines, younger and older ages at treatment, and gender.

## DISCUSSION

The relationship between cumulative anthracycline dose and subsequent cardiac problems is complex and a function of many different factors. This study points to cumulative dose, gender, and age at irradiation as three important independent variables. The resulting model is fairly predictive of those who will have good or poor exercise test outcomes, although there is considerable room for improvement.

Why gender is an important factor remains unclear. Females were more likely to have abnormally low ejection fractions or cardiac indices than their male counterparts, after adjusting for cumulative dose of anthracycline and age at treatment. The possibility that the normal ranges defined in our study were inappropriate for females seems unlikely. We used standard body surface area indexing to determine normal ranges for all patients undergoing exercise ergometry, and there should not be gender differences in cardiac output after indexing by body surface area. Furthermore, the cut-points for the low end of normal used in our cardiopulmonary exercise lab were almost identical between male and female controls. This coincides with other reports that have shown no difference between normal males and females with respect to cardiac output after indexing for body surface area and no gender differences in ejection fraction [18]. Consequently, we believe there was a real difference in outcome between the males and females in our study. Another possibility to explain this finding was that females in this study were more "out of condition" than their male counterparts. Possibly there are differences between sexes with respect to physical activity during and after cancer treatment, and therefore girls tested worse than boys. Still another possibility is that females are more at risk for cardiac damage than males, either because their hearts are in some way more susceptible to anthracyclines or because they may have a different metabolism or volume of distribution for anthracyclines than males. It is recognized that doxorubicin does not achieve high concentrations in fat and that obesity has been shown to slow the metabolism of doxorubicin [19]. If females of the same body surface area have more fat than males, and if anthracyclines do not distribute into fat, then equivalent meter-squared doses may lead to higher concentrations of anthracycline in the hearts of females than males. Since gender differences in body composition are more apparent in children postpubertal than prepubertal, we also analyzed the logistic regression model between children under 12 years versus those 12 or older. The model showed an even greater relative risk of test abnormalities in older girls than older boys. The relative risk associated with female gender in children 12 years or older at treatment was 5.1 (95% confidence interval, 17.9, 1.5). This effect was larger than the overall relative risk for female gender as compared to male gender, which was 3.1 (6.3, 1.5), using all children. Hrushesky et al. [20] have reported

an imbalance in the ratio of adult men to women who developed anthracycline-induced congestive heart failure (CHF), with 1 of 10 males developing CHF as compared to 7 of 24 females. This imbalance may have been due to differing disease states and anthracycline doses (80% of the males had bladder cancer and received a mean dose of 474 mg/m$^2$ of doxorubicin, whereas the women predominantly had ovarian cancer and received a mean dose of 516 mg/m$^2$ of doxorubicin). No formal analysis was conducted to sort out these confounding variables, and thus Hrushesky et al. did not conclude that a gender effect was present.

The dose-response curve for anthracyclines is also of interest. The probabilities associated with adverse outcome are, as one would expect, much higher with exercise testing than with CHF as an outcome measure. Age and gender appear to have a major role in these probability estimates. Of interest, heart irradiation did not significantly affect these results. This may have been true for a number of reasons. Most likely, the radiation therapy effect was not large enough for us to detect in this study. Furthermore, the measures of heart irradiation exposure did not include a more comprehensive dose–volume analysis that would have required computerized tomographic radiation treatment planning, not available for this study. Possibly the time of follow-up was not long enough to see the irradiation effect, although we looked for but saw no direct evidence for this.

The importance of our findings rests on the increased awareness of the nonlethal toxicity associated with anthracyclines. Quantifying and displaying the risks of this undesirable side effect of treatment makes it possible to incorporate these risks into our decision-making process more precisely. The risks of every added dose of an anthracycline must be weighed against the expected benefit to be derived [9]. When the perceived benefits are relatively small, then the predicted risk of the nonlethal adverse outcomes we describe in this report must be seriously considered. Furthermore, we do not yet know if the abnormal findings we report here are a harbinger of more serious problems (including CHF) in the future.

In summary, we have shown a significant association between cumulative anthracycline dose and abnormal cardiac function as measured by the tests we used. We also found that age and gender are additional factors, with younger age at treatment and female gender associated with worse test outcomes [21]. These findings should help clinicians decide when the benefits of anthracycline outweigh their risks, and, in so doing, improve therapeutic decision making.

## ACKNOWLEDGMENTS

This work was funded in part by NIH Research Career Development Award KO4-CA01480, for which Dr. Silber was the recipient.

## REFERENCES

1. Von Hoff DD, Layard M, Basa P: Risk factors for doxorubicin induced congestive heart failure. Ann Intern Med 91:701–717, 1979.
2. Von Hoff DD, Rozencweig M, Layard M, et al.: Daunomycin-induced cardiotoxicity in children and adults. Am J Med 62:200–208, 1977.
3. Praga C, Beretta G, Vigo PL, et al.: Adriamycin cardiotoxicity: A survey of 1273 patients. Cancer Treat Rep 63:827–834, 1979.
4. Lipshultz SE, Colan SD, Gelber RD, et al.: Late cardiac effects of doxorubicin therapy for acute lymphoblastic leukemia in childhood. N Engl J Med 324:808–815, 1991.
5. Steinherz L, Steinherz P, Tan C, Heller G, Murphy L: Cardiac toxicity 4 to 20 years after completing anthracycline therapy. J Am Med Assoc 266:1672–1677, 1991.
6. Larsen RL, Jakacki RI, Vetter VL, Meadows AT, Silber JH, Barber G: Electrocardiographic changes and arrhythmias after cancer therapy in children and young adults. Am J Cardiol 70:73–77, 1992.
7. Clavell LA, Gelber RD, Cohen HJ, Hitchcock-Bryan S, Cassidy JR, Tarbell NJ, Blattner SR, Tantrawabi R, Leavitt P, Sallan SE: Four-agent induction and intensive asparaginase therapy for treatment of childhood acute lymphoblastic leukemia. N Engl J Med 315:657–663, 1986.
8. Santoro A, Bonadonna G, Valagussa P, et al.: Long-term results of combined chemotherapy–radiotherapy approach in Hodgkin's disease: Superiority of ABVD plus radiotherapy versus MOPP plus radiotherapy. J Clin Oncol 5:27–37, 1987.
9. Silber JH, Kaizer H: Marginal analysis applied to the dose–response curve. Med Pediat Oncol 16:344–348, 1988.
10. Jakacki RI, Goldwein JW, Larsen RL, Barber G, Silber JH: Cardiac dysfunction following spinal irradiation during childhood. J Clin Oncol 11:1033–1038, 1993.
11. Green MV, Ostrow MG, Douglas MA, et al.: High temporal resolution ECG gated scintigraphic angiocardiography. J Nucl Med 16:95, 1975.
12. Alexander J, Dainiak N, Berger HJ, et al.: Serial assessment of doxorubicin cardiotoxicity with quantitative radionuclide angiocardiography. N Engl J Med 300:278–283, 1979.
13. Palmeri ST, Bonow RO, Myers CE, et al.: Prospective evaluation of doxorubicin cardiotoxicity by rest and exercise radionuclide angiography. Am J Cardiol 58:607–613, 1986.
14. James FW, Kaplan S, Glueck C, et al.: Responses of normal children and young adults to controlled bicycle exercise. Circulation 61:902–912, 1980.
15. Tanner CS, Heise CT, Barber G: Correlation of the physiologic parameters of a continuous ramp versus an incremental James exercise protocol in normal children. Am J Cardiol 67:309–312, 1991.
16. Triebwasser JH, Johnson RL, Burpo RP, et al.: Noninvasive determination of cardiac output by a modified acetylene rebreathing procedure utilizing mass spectrometer measurements. Aviation Space Environ Med 48:203–209, 1977.
17. Kallay MC, Hyde RW, Smith RJ, et al.: Cardiac output by rebreathing in patients with cardiopul-

monary diseases. J Appl Physiol 63:201–210, 1987.

18. Sullivan MJ, Cobb FR, Higginbotham MB: Stroke volume increases by similar mechanisms during upright exercise in normal men and women. Am J Cardiol 67:1405–1412, 1991.

19. Rodvold KA, Rushing DA, Tewksbury DA: Doxorubicin clearance in the obese. J Clin Oncol 6:1321–1327, 1988.

20. Hrushesky JM, Darrell JF, Berestka JS, et al.: Diminishment of respiratory sinus arrythmia forshadows doxorubicin-induced cardiomyopathy. Circulation 84:697–707, 1991.

21. Silber JH, Jakacki R, Larson R, Barber G: Forcasting exercise function after anthracyclines in childhood: The role of dose, age and sex. Proc ASCO 11:370 (abstr 1280), 1992.

# 11. The Use of the Corrected QT Interval (QT$_c$) in Screening for Anthracycline-Related Cardiotoxicity

Cindy L. Schwartz, M.D., Susie S. Truesdell, P.A., and Edward B. Clark, M.D.

Oncologists have been able to maximize the therapeutic benefit of anthracyclines while minimizing the likelihood of acute cardiotoxicity by consideration of the patient's cumulative anthracycline dosage and by monitoring cardiac function [1,2]. Subclinical myocardial damage resulting from anthracyclines was not considered to be a problem until recently, when reports of late-onset cardiomyopathy and cardiac dysrhythmia began to appear [3,4]. As a result of the aggressive use of anthracyclines, a large contingent of patients have survived free of cancer. Having received what appeared to be maximally tolerated doses of anthracyclines, they now appear to be at risk for late cardiac decompensation.

Identification of those patients at greatest risk of late cardiac decompensation is essential if interventions to maintain clinical well-being are to be devised. There is a justifiable reluctance to routinely subject clinically well individuals to a large battery of costly and sometimes invasive cardiac testing, in the absence of factors known to be predictive of late manifestations. We therefore used an alternative approach. Resting electrocardiograms (ECG) and two-dimensional echocardiograms (ECHO) were evaluated for subtle abnormalities of measurements known to become abnormal in acute anthracycline-induced cardiomyopathy [5,6]. Such measurements include the fractional shortening (FS) and corrected QT interval (QT$_c$). Further cardiac evaluation was reserved for those with definite abnormalities in either of these values.

## METHODS

A Follow-Up Clinic was established at the University of Rochester Medical Center in May 1988 to provide comprehensive multidisciplinary care of patients treated during childhood (age 21 years) for cancer. Patients involved in the clinic are: (1) more than 5 years from the time of initial diagnosis; (2) off cytotoxic therapy for more than 2 years; and (3) in complete remission. Patients undergo baseline screening of organs that may have been damaged by the particular cytotoxic regimen used. For example, those patients who had received anthracycline were advised to undergo a resting ECG and an ECHO in addition to the history and physical examination.

The QT$_c$ was calculated from the ECG by the following formula:

$$\frac{QT}{\sqrt{RR}}$$

(QT is the time in msec between the beginning of the Q wave and the end of the T wave. RR is the time between sequential R waves.) The QT and the corresponding RR intervals were measured for several complexes [4–8] on each ECG and the individual $QT_c$ values were averaged to determine the patient's $QT_c$. For those patients with more than one ECG performed, the most recent was used for analysis of the $QT_c$ data of the entire group.

FS was calculated from the echocardiogram as follows:

$$\frac{LVDD - LVSD}{LVDD} \times 100$$

LVDD = left ventricular diastolic dimension; LVSD = left ventricular systolic dimension.

Those patients whose ECGs were abnormal were advised to have electrocardiographic exercise testing. Exercises were performed on a bicycle ergometer according to the Godfrey protocol [7]. Each minute, the workload was increased by 10-, 15-, or 20-watt increments (determined by height). During exercise and recovery, the ECG and blood pressure were recorded each minute.

Cumulative anthracycline doses were calculated for all patients. One mg/m² of doxorubicin (1 ANTH) was considered to be equivalent in cardiotoxic potential to 1.5 mg/m² of daunorubicin. For those who were younger than age 2, actual doses in mg/kg were converted to mg/m² by the following formula: (mg/kg × 30 kg/m² = mg/m²). All patients were in remission at the time they were initially evaluated. None were sedated and none were receiving cardiac medication.

## RESULTS

Two hundred thirteen of 274 known surviving patients treated for childhood cancer between 1970 and 1987 and followed by the Division of Pediatric Hematology–Oncology at the University of Rochester have been evaluated in the four years that the Follow-Up Clinic has been in operation. Fifty-seven of these patients had been treated with ≥100 ANTH. Sixteen had radiation fields that included the heart. Resting ECHOs and ECGs were performed in six of nine patients who had received 100–199 ANTH (including one with cardiac irradiation) and 47 of 48 patients who had received 200–550 ANTH.

One patient who had received 300 ANTH and pulmonary radiation therapy had symptomatic congestive heart failure when evaluated in long-term clinic. Her $QT_c$ could not be measured adequately due to T-wave changes associated with ischemia; it is therefore not included in further analysis. However, from the time congestive heart failure was noted at the end of therapy until the ischemic changes were noted 6 years later, her $QT_c$ was between 0.45–0.47 on numerous ECGs. She has died of heart failure.

Figure 1 shows the percentage of patients receiving 100–199, 200–299, 300–399, and 400–550 ANTH (no chest irradiation) who had a $QT_c$ ≥0.43 and ≥0.45. Figure 2 is a similar analysis for all patients (± radiation). It is clear from these figures that the $QT_c$ prolongation occurs more frequently in patients who have received higher doses of ANTH.

Table 1 shows the statistical significance of these findings in both groups (without radiotherapy, all patients). Of those patients who did not have chest irradiation, 0 of 15 who received <300 ANTH versus 6 of 22 who received ≥300 ANTH had a $QT_c$ ≥0.45 (P = .03, Fischer's exact). Three of 15 who received <300 ANTH versus 12 of 22 who received ≥300 ANTH had a $QT_c$ ≥0.43 (P = .03). For all patients, 0 of 19 who received <300 ANTH versus 7 of 33 who received ≥300 ANTH had a $QT_c$ ≥0.45 (P = .03). Three of 19 who received <300 ANTH versus 19 of 33 who received ≥300 ANTH

# QTc vs. Dose

## No RT

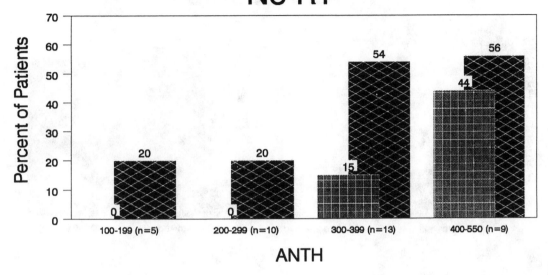

**Figure 1.**

**TABLE 1. QT$_c$ Versus Anthracycline Dose**

|       | QT$_c$ | <300 | ≥300 | P |
|-------|--------|------|------|------|
| No RT | ≥0.45  | 0/15 | 6/22 | .03 |
| No RT | ≥0.43  | 3/15 | 12/22 | .03 |
| All   | ≥0.45  | 0/19 | 7/33 | .03 |
| All   | ≥0.43  | 3/19 | 19/33 | .003 |

had a QT$_c$ of ≥0.43 (P = .003).

Seven patients who were initially seen in 1988 or 1989 have had follow-up ECGs. All four with QT$_c$ ≥0.43 have had further prolongation over the years. The three with initial QT$_c$ ≥0.42 have not.

All 52 patients had resting ECHOs. Only one patient with a history of congestive heart failure while on therapy 13 years earlier had an abnormal FS of 26% (normal ≥28%) and a QT$_c$ of 0.44. Having been treated for bilateral femoral osteosarcoma,

she was unable to perform exercise testing on the Godfrey bicycle. The incidence of FS in the low normal range was not significantly increased after ≥300 or ≥450 mg/m² of anthracycline. No other consistent abnormalities in the echocardiograms were noted in these patients.

Those with prolongation of the QT$_c$ were advised to undergo exercise ECG testing. Table 2 shows the results of these tests. Exercise testing was performed in three of five patients with an initial QT$_c$ of ≥0.45 (two patients had QT$_c$ ≥0.45 on later tests). Six with initial QT$_c$ of 0.42–0.44 also had exercise testing performed. The patients with QT$_c$ of 0.44–0.46 all had QT$_c$ prolongation with exercise, as did two of the patients with a QT$_c$ of 0.43. The other two patients with a QT$_c$ of 0.43 and the patient with a QT$_c$ of 0.42 had shortening of the QT$_c$ with exercise (normal).

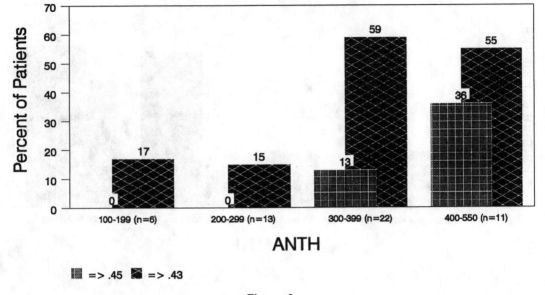

# QTc vs. Dose
## All Patients

ANTH

■ => .45   ▨ => .43

**Figure 2.**

## DISCUSSION

Subclinical cardiac damage induced by anthracycline therapy was initially thought to improve or remain stable with time [8]. The recent recognition of late cardiac decompensation in patients treated during childhood suggests that subclinical damage may progress with time, or that compensatory mechanisms that initially permit normal function may later become inadequate. Factors responsible for this late decompensation, and methods of intervention, can be determined when screening tests are available that recognize persistent cardiac injury.

The cardiac risks for long-term survivors of childhood cancer who received anthracyclines include congestive heart failure and sudden death by arrhythmia [3,4]. The $QT_c$ is of particular interest be-cause it may suggest risk for either arrhythmia or heart failure. Congenital prolongation of the QT interval predisposes the child to arrhythmias and sudden death [9]. Bender et al. described prolongation of the $QT_c$ interval during anthracycline therapy in children [6]. Those patients whose $QT_c$ interval was in excess of 0.46 progressed to cardiac failure within one or two more doses of anthracycline. A $QT_c$ >0.46 was associated with decreased FS [6].

We found, as did Bender et al., that prolongation of the $QT_c$ occurred more frequently in those patients who had received higher cumulative doses of anthracycline. The normal $QT_c$ interval is 0.40 ± .02. Those with $QT_c$ ≥0.45 are more than two standard deviations beyond the norm. This degree of $QT_c$ prolongation was seen more often in our patients re-

**TABLE 2.  Effects of Exercise on the QT$_c$**

| Patient/TX[a] | Initial QT$_c$ | Prolongation | Exercise Tolerance |
|---|---|---|---|
| TU 460 | 0.46 | 0.05 | Poor |
| LA 450 | 0.46 | 0.02 | Poor |
| JM 305 + TBI[a] | 0.45 | 0.04 | Normal |
| GT 550 | 0.44 | 0.05 | Not done |
| KL 355 + lung | 0.43 | 0.05 | Poor |
| KS 175 | 0.43 | 0.04 | Not done |
| MM 321 | 0.43 | No (-.09) | Normal |
| JN 295 | 0.43 | No (-.08) | Normal |
| KJ 480 | 0.42 | No (-.04) | Poor |

[a]TX, therapy; TBI, total body irradiations.

ceiving ≥300 ANTH. In addition, more patients with a QT$_c$ ≥0.43 (more than one standard deviation beyond the mean) had received ≥300 ANTH. This is consistent with our expectation that more patients treated with higher cumulative doses would experience persistent cardiac injury compared with those who had received lower doses.

We do not yet know whether QT$_c$ prolongation will identify those long-term survivors whose cardiac injury will progress with time. QT$_c$ measurements in the majority of our patients from the time of their treatment are not available. We cannot determine whether the prolonged QT$_c$ intervals noted herein reflect persistent or progressive damage. It is, however, of concern that all four patients with an initial QT$_c$ ≥0.43 retested 2–3 years later have had further QT$_c$ prolongation, while three patients with QT$_c$ ≥0.42 have not had further prolongation.

The QT$_c$ interval normally becomes shorter during exercise [10]. However, in those individuals with known congenital prolonged QT syndrome (and the associated risk of arrhythmias), the QT$_c$ interval becomes longer during maximal exercise [11]. Patients with normal QT$_c$ intervals, but episodes of syncope provoked by stress, have also been reported to have prolongation of the QT$_c$ with exercise [12].

All four patients tested with a QT$_c$ of ≥0.44 showed prolongation of the QT$_c$ with exercise. This may be indicative of a risk of sudden arrhythmias and death. One of these four patients has reported syncopal events. Holter monitoring of this patient showed occasional episodes of sinus tachycardia and occasional sinus arrhythmias resulting in sinus bradycardia.

The QT$_c$ interval is one of the few cardiac tests that an oncologist can easily gain the expertise to read. (For accurate results, it is essential that the RR associated with the given QT duration be measured and that values obtained from several complexes be averaged.) Asymptomatic patients who received ≥200 ANTH now are advised to have annual ECGs with ECHOs every 3 years. Further evaluation is performed for prolongation of the QT$_c$ interval to ≥0.45 (in patients who are in normal electrolyte balance and on no medication), a decrease in QRS voltage, significant T-wave changes, clinical symptoms, or a decrease in FS. Annual QT$_c$ measurement may assure the timely detection of those with myocardial injury and may enable us to note progressive change easily. Exercise testing may facilitate the detection and evaluation of cardiac injury caused by anthracycline therapy. Further evaluation is necessary to

determine the predictive value of a prolonged $QT_c$.

## REFERENCES

1. Lefrak EA, Pitha J, Rosenheim S, Gottlieb JA: A clinico-pathologic analysis of Adriamycin cardiotoxicity. Cancer 32:302–314, 1973.

2. Ritchfie JL, Singer JW, Thorning D, Sorensen SG, Hamilton GW: Anthracycline cardiotoxicity: Clinical and pathologic outcomes assessed by radionuclide ejection fraction. Cancer 46:1109–1116, 1980.

3. Steinherz L, Steinherz P, Tan C, Heller G, Murphy L: Cardiac toxicity 4 to 20 years after completing anthracycline therapy. J Am Med Assoc 266:1672–1677, 1991.

4. Steinherz L, Steinherz P: Delayed cardiac toxicity from anthracycline therapy. Pediatrician 18:49–52, 1991.

5. Lewis AB, Pilkington R, Rakahashi M, et al.: Echocardiographic assessment of anthracycline cardiotoxic-ity in children. Med Pediatr Oncol 5:167, 1978.

6. Bender KS, Shematek JP, Leventhal BG, Kan JS: QT interval prolongation associated with anthracycline cardiotoxicity. J Pediatr 105:442–444, 1984.

7. Godfrey S (ed): Exercise Testing in Children. Philadelphia: W.B. Saunders, 1974.

8. Goorin AM, Borow KM, Goldman A, Williams RG, Henderson IC, Sallan SE, Cohen HJ, Jaffe N: Congestive heart failure due to Adriamycin cardiotoxicity: Its natural history in children. Cancer 47:2810–2816, 1981.

9. Schwartz PJ, Periti M, Malliami A: The long QT syndrome. Am Heart J 89:378–390, 1975.

10. Bucsenez D, von Bernuth G: The QT interval during exercise in healthy children 6–14 years old. J Electrocardiol 22(1):17–19, 1989.

11. Van Gundy JC, Schaffer MS, Washington RL, Daberkow E, Wolfe RR: Effects of exercise in patients with known congenital prolonged QT syndrome. Am J Cardiol 60:14, 1987.

12. Phillips J, Ichinose H: Clinical and pathologic studies in the hereditary syndrome of a long QT interval, syncopal spells and sudden death. Chest 58(3):236–243, 1970.

# 12. Prevention of Cardiac Damage Due to Adriamycin: Modification of Method of Administration

Michael S. Ewer, M.D., M.P.H., and Robert S. Benjamin, M.D.

## HISTORICAL PERSPECTIVE

The anthracycline doxorubicin (Adriamycin) has been in our therapeutic armamentarium for two decades. The toxicities of this important agent became apparent during clinical trials and are still of vital concern. The most notable toxic effect observed during phase I studies was mucositis, which was more common when schedules utilizing frequently repeated drug administrations were used [1]. When pharmacokinetic studies revealed a long plasma half-life, it was recommended that Adriamycin be given according to an intermittent high-dose schedule administered as a rapid intravenous infusion and repeated every 3 weeks [2,3]. Such a schedule reduces mucositis to an acceptable level and has been widely implemented; it is still considered the standard schedule for Adriamycin administration.

Cardiotoxicity is a potentially life-threatening complication of Adriamycin therapy; the degree of cardiac damage was shown to be related to the cumulative dose. Weiss et al. [4] were the first to suggest a possible alteration in the cardiotoxic characteristics of Adriamycin with schedule modification. In their study, Adriamycin was given according to a weekly schedule, and decreased cardiac toxicity was noted. Decreased cardiotoxicity with weekly sched-

ules was confirmed by Chlebowski et al. [5]. Von Hoff et al. [6] emphasized the importance of administration schedules with regard to cardiotoxicity. They analyzed the data by life-table methodology and compared cumulative event-free survival, defined as freedom from congestive heart failure, and its reciprocal, cumulative incidence of congestive heart failure, with cumulative dose. By means of this analysis these investigators were able to demonstrate a highly significant difference between the cumulative incidence of congestive heart failure when the drug was given according to a weekly schedule compared with every-third-week administration. Gottlieb was the first to recognize the relationship of cumulative dose and the risk of cardiac toxicity with the standard schedule [7]. He proposed a cutoff cumulative dose of 600 mg/$m^2$, which was subsequently decreased to 550 mg/$m^2$, and 450 mg/$m^2$ [8,9].

Clinical experience has demonstrated considerable variability as to the maximum tolerated cumulative dose of Adriamycin, and more recent studies have suggested parameters based on cardiac structure, function, and clinical evaluation of the patient to help in deciding when to continue or when to stop the drug. Singer et al. [10] and Alexander et al. [11] demonstrated the importance of cardiac ejection fraction as measured by nuclear scanning techniques in monitoring cardiac function. Ultrastructural abnormalities associated with Adriamycin were reported by Billingham et al. [12] and Bristow et al. [13], who proposed a grading scale for Adriamycin toxicity. The ultrastructural changes are of special importance, as these changes can usually be found in patients before there is clinical evidence of cardiac dysfunction. Our studies, which use a modified grading scale proposed by Mackay et al. [14], indicate that a high endomyocardial biopsy grade (greater than 1.5) is the best predictor of increased risk of developing heart failure should therapy with Adriamycin or an Adriamycin-containing regimen be continued [15].

## CONTINUOUS INFUSION REGIMENS

A number of studies have confirmed lower levels of cardiotoxicity when Adriamycin is administered according to schedules that in some way distribute the total dose, thereby reducing the peaks in blood level that are otherwise produced. A number of such alternate schedules have been investigated: Valdivieso et al. [16] demonstrated statistically significant differences in mean biopsy grade when weekly versus 3-weekly Adriamycin was administered in a randomized study of 100 patients. For patients receiving the drug according to a weekly schedule, the mean biopsy grade was 0.46 (12 patients, 16 biopsies), while patients who received the drug according to the 3-weekly rapid infusion schedule had a mean biopsy grade of 1.39 (16 patients, 19 biopsies; $P = .01$). None of these patients experienced congestive heart failure, and five, all of whom received the drug by weekly schedule, exceeded a cumulative Adriamycin dose of 540 mg/m$^2$.

Torti et al. [17] reported similar results,

obtained in a series of 125 patients, 98 of whom received 3-weekly Adriamycin and the remaining 27 received the drug weekly. Patients receiving weekly Adriamycin were able to tolerate 168 mg/m$^2$ more Adriamycin than patients treated on the 3-weekly schedule for equivalent degrees of cardiac toxicity. Patients on a weekly schedule would be expected to tolerate an additional 2–4 months of an Adriamycin-containing regimen over what would be expected of patients treated on the 3-weekly schedule.

The most plausible explanation for the phenomenon of decreased cardiac toxicity of weekly Adriamycin compared with 3-weekly schedules is a reduction in peak plasma levels; the peak level from 1/3 of the dose is lower, and there is a longer period of time for elimination of the drug before the next dose is given. Simply dividing the dose over 3 days provides little or no cardiac protection [6]. The most practical way to reduce peak drug levels is to prolong infusion time.

A phase I study was initiated to evaluate any alteration in cardiotoxicity with prolongation of infusion time [18]. A fixed dose of 60 mg/m$^2$ was given with escalation of infusion time from 24 hours to 48 hours, and then to 96 hours. It had been anticipated that the dose-limiting toxicity would be mucositis, but at the 60 mg/m$^2$ dose, dose-limiting toxicity was not reached. Peak plasma levels decreased from 1.31 µg/ml when the drug was given by rapid infusion to 0.24, 0.13, and 0.10 µg/ml with 24-, 48-, and 96-hour infusions, respectively. We were greatly concerned that with a decrease in cardiotoxicity there might be a similar decrease in antitumor effect. A single-agent regimen of Adriamycin was studied in patients with metastatic breast cancer who had failed previous treatment with cyclophosphamide, methotrexate, and fluorouracil (CMF). A response rate of 50% was achieved, and we were able to conclude that efficacy had not been appreciably altered. Subsequent studies using combination chemotherapy in patients with sarcomas [19,20] and patients with metastatic breast cancer [21] confirmed that no interference with antitumor activity had taken place.

Evaluation of cardiac toxicity with prolonged infusion regimens demonstrated a significant decrease in the cardiac biopsy grades for patients treated by continuous infusion as opposed to rapid infusion [22]. The cardiac biopsy grade for patients treated with continuous infusion was significantly lower than that for patients treated with rapid infusion (mean 0.9 ± 0.73; median 0.5 vs. mean 1.6 ± 0.88; median 1.5; $P = .004$ by Mann Whitney test). In addition, the incidence of biopsies considered to be high-grade (≥1.5) was 17% after continuous infusion, compared with 55% after rapid infusion ($P = .0001$). These differences are especially pertinent when one considers that a higher cumulative dose of Adriamycin was given to patients treated by continuous infusion, compared with that of patients treated with rapid infusion (median 600 mg/m²; range 360–1,500 mg/m² vs. median 465 mg/m²; range 290–680; $P = .002$ by Mann Whitney test).

Increased mucositis with longer infusion durations was considered a significant problem, and we subsequently studied infusion durations shorter than 96 hours [23]. To emphasize cardiac toxicity, we included only patients whose cumulative Adriamycin dose was more than 500 mg/m², and, in order to assure that observed differences were related to Adriamycin rather than other etiologies, we excluded patients with known cardiac risk factors. Twenty-four-hour continuous infusion was significantly less cardiotoxic than rapid infusion in that equivalent cardiac toxicity was seen only after an additional 310 mg/m² of Adriamycin had been given. The median dose for the 11 patients treated by rapid infusion, all of whom had been screened at 450 mg/m² to receive additional Adriamycin, was 550 mg/m² (range 500–650), while the median dose for the 16 patients treated by 24-hour infusion was 860 mg/m² (range 520–1,080).

Similar results were demonstrated for cardiac biopsies, where an identical mean biopsy grade of 1.3 was noted for both groups. Forty-five percent of the patients in the rapid infusion group, compared with 40% for the 24-hour continuous infusion group, demonstrated high-grade biopsies. A slightly higher incidence of heart failure was noted in the rapid infusion group (18% vs. 13%), but a lower incidence of asymptomatic ejection fraction <50 was seen in the rapid infusion group (10% vs. 31%). Overall, the differences in cardiac function were not statistically significant. The effect of 24-hour infusion is similar or slightly greater than weekly rapid infusion. With 24-hour infusion, about 310 mg/m² more Adriamycin can be given than with standard administration every 3 weeks; with weekly administration, about 168 mg/m² more Adriamycin can be given than with standard administration every 3 weeks.

## FORTY-EIGHT- AND 96-HOUR REGIMENS

Patients treated with 48-hour and 96-hour continuous infusions demonstrated significantly less overall cardiac toxicity than was observed in patients who had received Adriamycin by weekly schedules or by 24-hour infusions. The highest mean biopsy grade was 0.8 for the 48-hour group, who had received a median of 700 mg/m² (range 530–920). This compared favorably with an almost identical biopsy grade of 0.9, but at a considerably higher median Adriamycin dose of 945 mg/m² (range 600–1,905) for the 96-hour group. A comparison of the cardiac toxicity profile for patients receiving 96-hour continuous infusion therapy, when compared with 3-weekly administration, suggests that nearly double the cumulative dose of Adriamycin can be tolerated while still achieving less cardiac toxicity. These findings were also confirmed for patients with cardiac risk factors.

When comparing the dose–toxicity relationship for 48-hour and 96-hour schedules, it was noted that at each cumulative dose, the incidence of high-grade biopsies was lower with 96-hour infusion than with 48-hour infusion [24]. High-grade biopsies predict development of congestive heart failure should additional Adriamycin be given, so these data indicate that 96-hour infusion of Adriamycin is less cardiotoxic than 48-hour infusions.

The advantage of continuous infusion schedules in decreasing high cardiac biopsy grade is reflected in the clinical setting as a decrease in the incidence of congestive heart failure. Hortobagyi et al. studied a group of patients receiving combination chemotherapy for metastatic breast cancer, which included patients both with and without cardiac risk factors and heart failure related at least in part to causes other than Adriamycin. They found a significant decrease in the cumulative incidence of congestive heart failure in those who had been treated with continuous infusion regimens ($P$ = .004) [21]. A 10% incidence of heart failure was observed in patients who received Adriamycin by rapid infusion at a cumulative dose level of 450 mg/m², while a 10% incidence of heart failure was not noted until the 770 mg/m² level in those treated by 48–96-hour continuous infusions. None of the 70 patients without pre-existing risk factors who were treated with continuous infusion Adriamycin developed congestive heart failure, while 5 of 71 treated with rapid infusions experienced this complication.

The longer the period of infusion up to 96 hours, the lower the cardiac toxicity. These data strongly suggest that peak plasma levels of Adriamycin play a pivotal role in the production of cardiomyopathy. The only previously known peak-level toxicities of Adriamycin were true bolus effects: facial flushing, hypotension, and occasional anaphylactoid reactions [1]. It is now clear from these studies that cardiac toxicity is also peak-level related; additionally, nausea and vomiting decreased in direct proportion to decreasing peak levels and thus can also be considered peak-level phenomena. Antitumor efficacy and myelosuppression are unchanged by schedule alteration, and are probably related to overall drug exposure as approximated by the integral, rather than by the peak, of the plasma disappearance curve. In contrast, mucositis appears to be dependent on the duration of exposure. Combination of cardioprotective agents with 24- or 48-hour infusions may permit further decrease in cardiac toxicity without an increase in mucositis.

## CONCLUSION

It is difficult to demonstrate that higher cumulative Adriamycin doses can improve survival. It is clear nevertheless that some patients may benefit from additional therapy. Patients continuing to respond and who are in near-complete remission when standard dose limitations are reached, or those who relapse late with sensitive tumors, are examples of those who can benefit from higher cumulative doses. In the previously noted study of breast cancer patients [21], the duration of complete remission was prolonged by 8 months, compared with that of patients treated with standard regimens ($P$ = .15). This extension approximates the duration of additional Adriamycin therapy given those patients.

Ideally, the duration of therapy should be determined on the basis of tumor control strategies rather than on arbitrary limitations for cardiac toxicity. Even if the recommended cumulative doses for an oncologic entity are modest, there is no need to use methods shown to be more cardiotoxic in reaching those levels. They may prevent the drug's continuation or reutilization in an appropriate patient should it be needed at a later time. As Adriamycin is increasingly used in the treatment of curable patients, long-term complications as well as the potential for drug utilization in treatment of a secondary neoplasm must be taken into account in planning primary therapy. There is decreasing justification for continuing the more toxic regimen of rapid Adriamycin infusion.

## REFERENCES

1. Benjamin RS: A practical approach to Adriamycin (NSC 123127) toxicology. Cancer Chemother Rep 6:191–194, 1975.
2. Benjamin RS, Riggs CE Jr, Bachur NR: Pharmacokinetics and metabolism of Adriamycin in man. Clin Pharmacol Ther 14:592–600, 1973.
3. Benjamin RS, Wiernik PH, Bachur NR: Adriamycin chemotherapy—efficacy, safety, and pharmacologic basis of an intermittent single high-dosage schedule. Cancer 33:19–27, 1974.
4. Weiss AJ, Metter GE, Fletcher WS, Wilson WL, Grage TB, Ramirez G: Studies on Adriamycin using a weekly regimen demonstrating its clinical effectiveness and lack of cardiac toxicity. Cancer Treat Rep 60:813–822, 1976.
5. Chlebowski RT, Paroly WS, Pugh RP, Hueser J, Jacobs WM, Pajak TF, Bateman JR: Adriamycin given as a weekly schedule without a loading course: Clinically effective with reduced incidence of cardiotoxicity. Cancer Treat Rep 64:47–51, 1980.
6. Von Hoff DD, Layard MW, Basa P, Davis HL Jr, Von Hoff AL, Rozencweig M, Muggia FM: Risk factors for doxorubicin-induced congestive heart failure. Ann Intern Med 91:710, 1979.
7. Gottlieb JA, Lefrak EA, O'Bryan RM, Burgess MA: Fatal Adriamycin cardiomyopathy (CMY)—prevention by dose limitation. Proc Am Assoc Cancer Res 14:89, 1973 (abstr).
8. Lefrak EA, Pitha J, Rosenheim S, Gottlieb JA: A clinicopathologic analysis of Adriamycin cardiotoxicity. Cancer 32:302–314, 1973.
9. Minow RA, Benjamin RS, Lee ET, Gottlieb JA: Adriamycin cardiomyopathy risk factors. Cancer 39:1397–1402, 1977.
10. Singer JW, Narahara KA, Ritchie JL, Hamilton GW, Kennedy JW: Time- and dose-dependent changes in ejection fraction determined by radionuclide angiography after anthracycline therapy. Cancer Treat Rep 62:945–948, 1978.
11. Alexander J, Dainiak N, Berger HJ, Goldman L, Johnstone D, Reduto L, Duffy T, Schwartz P, Gottschalk A, Zaret BL: Serial assessment of doxorubicin cardiotoxicity with quantitative radionuclide angiocardiography. N Engl J Med 300:278–283, 1979.
12. Billingham ME, Bristow MR, Glastein E, Mason JW, Mason MA, Daniels JR: Adriamycin cardiotoxicity: Endomyocardial biopsy evidence of enhancement by irradiation. Am J Surg Path 1:17–23, 1977.
13. Bristow MR, Mason JW, Billingham ME, Daniels JR: Doxorubicin cardiomyopathy: Evaluation by phonocardiography, endomyocardial biopsy, and cardiac catheterization. Ann Intern Med 88:168–175, 1978.
14. Mackay B, Keyes LM, Benjamin RS, Ewer MS, Legha SS, Wallace S: Cardiac biopsy. TSEMJ (Texas Society for Electron Microscopy) 11:7–15, 1981.
15. Chawla SP, Benjamin RS, Legha SS, Ewer MS, Ali MK, Mackay B, Carrasco CH, Hortobagyi GN, Wallace S, Haynie III TP, Freireich EJ: Role of cardiac biopsy and radionuclide scans in monitoring of Adriamycin-induced cardiotoxicity. In Spitzy KH, Karrer K (eds): 13th International Congress of Chemotherapy. Vienna: Verlag H. Egermann, 1983, pp 490–492.
16. Valdivieso M, Burgess MA, Ewer MS, Mackay B, Wallace S, Benjamin RS, Ali MK, Bodey GP, Freireich EJ: Increased therapeutic index of weekly doxorubicin in the therapy of non-small cell lung cancer: A prospective, randomized study. J Clin Oncol 2:207–214, 1984.
17. Torti FM, Bristow MR, Howes AE, Aston D, Stocdale FE, Carter SK, Kohler M, Brown BW, Billingham ME: Reduced cardiotoxicity of doxorubicin delivered on a weekly schedule: Assessment by endomyocardial biopsy. Ann Intern Med 99:745–749, 1983.
18. Legha SS, Benjamin RS, Mackay B, Ewer M, Wallace S, Valdivieso M, Rasmussen SL, Blumenschein GR, Freireich EJ: Reduction of doxorubicin cardiotoxicity by prolonged continuous intravenous infusion. Ann Intern Med 96:133–139, 1982.

19. Benjamin RS, Yap BS: Infusion chemotherapy for soft tissue sarcomas. In Baker LH (ed): Soft Tissue Sarcoma. Amsterdam: Martinus Nijhoff, 1983, pp 109–115.

20. Benjamin RS, Murray JA, Carrasco CH, Raymond AK, Chawla SP, Wallace S, Ayala A, Papadopoulos NEJ, Plager C, Romsdahl MM: Preoperative chemotherapy for osteosarcoma: A treatment approach facilitating limb salvage with major prognostic implications. In Jones SE, Salmon SE (eds): Adjuvant Therapy of Cancer, vol 4. New York: Grune & Stratton, 1984, pp 601–610.

21. Hortobagyi GN, Frye D, Buzdar AU, Ewer MS, Fraschini G, Huy U, Ames F, Montague E, Carrasco CH, Mackay B, Benjamin RS: Decreased cardiac toxicity of doxorubicin administered by continuous intravenous infusion in combination chemotherapy for metastatic breast carcinoma. Cancer 63:37–45, 1989.

22. Legha SS, Benjamin RS, Mackay B, Yap HY, Wallace S, Ewer M, Blumenschein GR, Freireich EJ: Adriamycin therapy by continuous intravenous infusion in patients with metastatic breast cancer. Cancer 49:1762–1766, 1982.

23. Benjamin RS, Chawla SP, Hortobagyi GN, Ewer MS, Mackay B, Legha SS, Carrasco H, Wallace S: Continuous-infusion Adriamycin. In Rosenthal CJ, Rotman M (eds): Clinical Applications of Continuous Infusion Chemotherapy and Concomitant Radiation Therapy. New York: Plenum Press, 1986, pp 19–25.

24. Benjamin RS, Chawla SP, Ewer MS, Hortobagyi GN, Mackay B, Legha SS, Carrasco CH, Wallace S: Adriamycin cardiac toxicity and assessment of approaches to cardiac monitoring and cardioprotection. In Hatcher MP, Lazo JS, Tritton TR (eds): Organ Directed Toxicities of Anticancer Drugs. Boston: Martinus Nijhoff Publishing, 1988, pp 41–55.

# 13. The Use of Cardioprotectant Agents in Combination With Anthracycline Chemotherapy

Stacey L. Berg, M.D., Frank M. Balis, M.D., Linda McClure, R.N., David G. Poplack, M.D., and Marc E. Horowitz, M.D.

The anthracyclines are among the most active anticancer agents in the current armamentarium. Daunomycin is an integral part of the induction regimens for both acute lymphoblastic leukemia and acute nonlymphoblastic leukemia, while doxorubicin is a mainstay of therapy for pediatric and adult solid tumors. Unfortunately, treatment with anthracyclines also conveys the risk of one of the most devastating complications of anticancer therapy, potentially fatal cardiac toxicity.

The cardiotoxicity associated with anthracyclines has been recognized since the early 1970s [1–3]. Although acute cardiotoxicity in the form of arrhythmias or myocarditis may occur, a more significant problem is chronic cardiac toxicity that may lead to congestive heart failure and death. The pathological changes found on endomyocardial biopsy specimens from patients treated with anthracyclines include myofibrillar loss, cytoplasmic vacuolization, and dilation of the sarcoplasmic reticulum [4,5]. The relationship between this form of cardiotoxicity and the cumulative anthracycline dose administered has been clearly established. Although anthracycline-related congestive heart failure may occur after cumulative doses as low as 100 mg/m$^2$, the incidence of drug-induced cardiomyopathy increases steeply

starting at a total dose of 500–550 mg/m$^2$ (or less if the patient has received mediastinal irradiation) [4–6]. For this reason, many current treatment regimens include a predetermined limit to the total planned anthracycline dose, as well as serial measurements of cardiac function.

The biochemical basis for anthracycline-mediated cardiac toxicity has now been identified. Anthracyclines are capable of undergoing single electron reduction in the hydroxyquinone moiety of chromophore ring structure (Fig. 1). The free radical species generated in this process may react with membrane lipids, causing oxidative damage to myocardial cells [7]. Such damage has been observed in the cell membrane, the mitochondrial membrane,

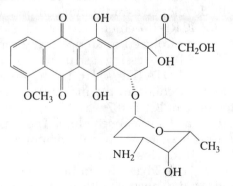

**Fig. 1.** The structure of doxorubicin.

*Cardiac Toxicity After Treatment for Childhood Cancer, pages 115–120, ©1993 Wiley-Liss, Inc.*

and the sarcoplasmic reticulum [8]. Although free radical formation can occur in other tissues, the heart has low levels of catalase, an enzyme that detoxifies free radicals, and is therefore particularly susceptible to free radical–induced damage [9].

The elucidation of the biochemical mechanism of anthracycline cardiotoxicity has led to the search for biochemical modulators of free radical reactions. Various free radical scavengers, such as N-acetyl cysteine and vitamin E (α-tocopherol), have shown promise in in vitro systems and some animal models, but none has demonstrated protection from anthracycline-induced cardiac damage in clinical trials [10–12].

The failure of free radical scavengers to reduce cardiac toxicity led to further examination of the role of iron in anthracycline-mediated free radical generation. Anthracyclines chelate iron (Fig. 2) with an affinity similar to that of desferroxamine [7]. The doxorubicin–iron complex catalyzes formation of extremely reactive hydroxyl radicals at the site of binding of the complex to membrane, implicating the complex in the development of cardiotoxicity [13].

Subsequently, the ability of iron chelators to protect against anthracycline cardiac toxicity was investigated. ICRF-159 (razoxane) and its soluble enantiomer ICRF-187 (Fig. 3) are chelating agents originally developed as antitumor compounds [14,15]. ICRF-187 enters cells by diffusion, then is hydrolyzed to an open-ring form (ICRF-198) possessing a structure similar to that of EDTA (Fig. 4) [16,17]. In phase I studies in children, the maximum tolerated dose of ICRF-187 was 3,500 mg/m²/day on a daily × 3 schedule. The dose-limiting toxicity was hepatic dysfunction, although myelosuppression was also observed [18]. Phase II studies, however, failed to demonstrate efficacy against pediatric malignancies [19].

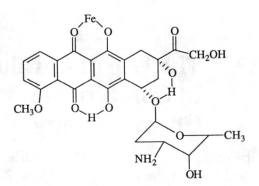

**Fig. 2.** The doxorubicin–iron complex.

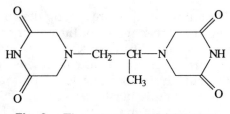

**Fig. 3.** The structure of ICRF-187.

Both ICRF-187 and ICRF-198 have been shown to remove iron from doxorubicin–iron complexes in vitro [20]. In the rat heart myocyte model, incubation with ICRF-187 both increases survival in the presence of doxorubicin and ameliorates doxorubicin-associated morphologic change [17]. Furthermore, in a variety of animal models, the administration of ICRF-187 in conjunction with doxorubicin has been demonstrated to protect both against morphologic evidence of myocardial damage and against clinical evidence of cardiomyopathy [12,21–24]. Protection is optimal when ICRF-187 is administered less than 2 hours before the doxorubicin dose [25] and when the ratio of ICRF-187 to doxorubicin is at least 10:1 [24]. Importantly, in vitro studies have shown no evidence of ICRF-187 protection of tumor cells from doxorubicin cytotoxicity, and, in fact, some evidence of synergy has been noted [26,27].

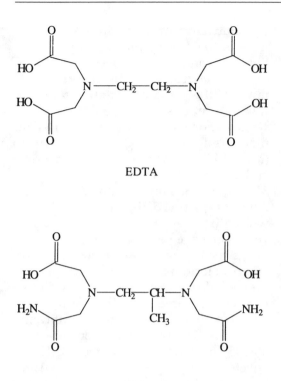

EDTA

ICRF-198

**Fig. 4.**  EDTA and ICRF-198.

Two approaches have been taken to evaluate the clinical efficacy of ICRF-187 cardioprotection. In a landmark study [28,29], Speyer et al. investigated whether the use of ICRF-187 could increase the total doxorubicin dose that could be safely administered. In this study, 150 women with advanced breast cancer were randomized to receive chemotherapy with either fluorouracil, doxorubicin, and cyclophosphamide alone (FDC) or the same regimen with ICRF-187. doxorubicin was administered as a bolus of 50 mg/m². ICRF-187 was administered at a dose of 1,000 mg/m² (a ratio of 20:1 to the doxorubicin dose) over 15 minutes, 30 minutes prior to doxorubicin. Treatment was continued until disease progression or limiting toxicity developed. Importantly, there was no predetermined upper limit to the cumulative doxorubicin

dose. Instead, the cardiologic criteria for stopping treatment included a fall in the resting left ventricular ejection fraction (LVEF) to less than 0.45, more than a 0.20 fall in LVEF from baseline, or a biopsy score of 2 or above.

Several important conclusions were drawn from this study. The response rates, progression-free survival, and overall survival were not statistically different in the two groups, suggesting that ICRF-187 did not antagonize the anticancer effect of doxorubicin. Furthermore, although the ICRF-187-treated group has a statistically greater degree of myelosuppression than the FDC-alone group, this did not appear to be of clinical significance. Other noncardiac toxicities also did not appear to differ between the two groups. Most importantly, this study showed a definite cardioprotective effect of ICRF-187 treatment. Two patients in the ICRF-187 arm had clinical congestive heart failure, compared with 20 in the control group, and only five of the ICRF-187-treated patients had a decrease in LVEF to <45% or a more than 20-point fall from baseline, compared with 32 patients in the control group. The mean decrease in LVEF was less in the ICRF-187 than in the FDC-alone arm for all ranges of total cumulative doxorubicin administration. In addition, ICRF-187 allowed the administration of significantly greater cumulative doses of doxorubicin: 26 patients in the ICRF-187 arm received a total doxorubicin dose greater than 700 mg/m², including 11 who received over 1,000 mg/m². This contrasted sharply with the FDC-alone group, in which only three patients received 700 mg/m² or more.

The results of this important study demonstrate that ICRF-187 administered prior to doxorubicin is protective and may allow many patients to receive a higher cumulative anthracycline dose than they would otherwise tolerate. In those patients who have had a good response to anthracycline therapy but who, because of the risk of cardiac toxicity, would previously have had to discontinue that therapy after receiving a predefined total anthracycline dose, administration of ICRF-187 may permit longer treatment with an effective agent. In addition, although not directly addressed in the Speyer study, the use of ICRF-187 also has the potential to enhance dose intensity of doxorubicin, for instance, by permitting higher individual doxorubicin doses while not requiring a concomitant reduction in the total number of doses administered.

Another approach to the evaluation of ICRF-187 is to determine whether its use in combination with a fixed total dose of doxorubicin will result in a decrease in the cardiotoxicity with that dose. Instead of attempting to maximize the total cumulative anthracycline dose that can be delivered, the object is to minimize cardiac toxicity observed with a fixed, "standard" cumulative dose. This strategy may be particularly important in children because they are at greater risk for the onset of cardiomyopathy many years after anthracycline therapy [30–32]. This approach to the use of ICRF-187 is being evaluated in a randomized prospective study in the Pediatric Branch of the National Cancer Institute.

In this protocol for the treatment of sarcoma patients with poor prognostic factors, chemotherapy consists of vincristine, doxorubicin, and cyclophosphamide alternating with etoposide and ifosfamide every 3 weeks for a total of 18 cycles. doxorubicin is administered as a 15-minute infusion. For the first three cycles, the dose is 35 mg/m$^2$/day for 2 days. For the remaining cycles, the dose is 50 mg/m$^2$/day on day 1 only. The total planned doxorubicin dose is 410 mg/m$^2$.

Based on the results from a pilot study of this regimen, the likelihood of patients' having an LVEF of less than 45% at a cumulative doxorubicin dose of 410 mg/m$^2$ was 40%. In the present protocol, patients are randomized to receive ICRF-187 or not. The drug is administered as a 15-minute infusion immediately prior to the doxorubicin dose, and the ratio of ICRF-187 to doxorubicin (in mg) is 20:1. LVEF is measured by multigated acquisition (MUGA) scan prior to the start of therapy and at a cumulative dose of 210 mg/m$^2$, 310 mg/m$^2$, 360 mg/m$^2$, and 410 mg/m$^2$. After completion of therapy, MUGA scans will be obtained three times in the first year, then once yearly.

The major objectives of this study are (1) to determine whether ICRF-187 can prevent doxorubicin-induced cardiotoxicity as measured by LVEF, (2) to determine whether ICRF-187 adds significantly to the toxicity of the treatment regimen, and (3) to determine whether ICRF-187 affects the efficacy of the regimen. Additional objectives include determination of the pharmacokinetic behavior of ICRF-187 in this group of pediatric patients and measurement of its effect on urinary excretion of iron and other metals.

Forty patients will be entered to achieve an 80% power to detect a difference of 12% in LVEF. So far, 37 patients have been entered. It is still too early to determine any cardioprotective benefit of ICRF-187. It does not appear, however, that ICRF-187 adds to the morbidity of the chemotherapy regimen in terms of an increased infection rate or any other clinical evidence of toxicity.

Anthracycline-based chemotherapy, despite its inherent toxicities, is likely to remain a mainstay of the treatment of pediatric malignancy for the foreseeable future. As the success rate of treatment increases, the long-term sequelae of therapy will assume increasing importance. Because cardiac toxicity obviously compromises both quality of life and survival, the development of strategies to reduce this toxicity is likely to remain an important area of both bench and clinical research. The use of ICRF-187 in conjunction with anthracyclines appears to be one promising approach to this difficult problem.

## REFERENCES

1. Lefrak E, Pitha J, Rosenheim S, et al.: A clinicopathologic analysis of Adriamycin cardiotoxicity. Cancer 32:302–314, 1973.
2. Gilladoga A, Manuel C, Tan C, et al.: The cardiotoxicity of Adriamycin and daunomycin in children. Cancer 37:1070–1078, 1976.
3. Halazun J, Wagner H, Gaeta J, et al.: Daunorubicin cardiac toxicity in children with acute lymphocytic leukemia. Cancer 33:545–553, 1974.
4. Bristow M, Mason J, Billingham M, et al.: Dose–effect and structure–function relationships in doxorubicin cardiomyopathy. Am Heart J 102:709–718, 1981.
5. Ferrans V: Overview of cardiac pathology in relation to anthracycline cardiotoxicity. Cancer Treat Rep 62:955–961, 1978.
6. Von Hoff D, Layard M, Basa P, et al.: Risk factors for doxorubicin-induced congestive heart failure. Ann Intern Med 91:710–717, 1979.
7. Myers C, Chabner B: Anthracyclines. In B Chabner, J Collins (eds): Cancer Chemotherapy: Principles and Practice. Philadelphia: JB Lippincott, 1990, pp 356–381.
8. Doroshow J: Effect of anthracycline antibiotics on oxygen radical formation in rat heart. Cancer Res 43:460–473, 1983.
9. Doroshow J, Locker G, Meyers C: Enzymatic defenses of the mouse heart against reactive oxygen metabolites: Alterations produced by doxorubicin. J Clin Invest 65:128–135, 1980.
10. Legha S, Wang Y-M, Mackay B, et al.: Clinical and pharmacologic investigation of the effects of alpha-tocopherol on Adriamycin cardiotoxicity. Proc NY Acad Sci pp 411–418, 1982.
11. Doroshow J, Locker G, Ifrim I, et al.: Prevention of doxorubicin cardiac toxicity in the mouse by N-acetylcysteine. J Clin Invest 68:1053–1064, 1981.
12. Herman E, Ferrars V, Meyers C, et al.: Comparison of the effectiveness of (-/+-1,2-bis(3,5 dioxopiiperazinyl-yl)propane (ICRF-187) and N-acetycysteine in preventing chronic doxorubicin cardiotoxicity in beagles. Cancer Res 45:276–281, 1985.
13. Myers C, Gianni L, Simone C, et al.: Oxidative destruction of erythrocyte ghost membranes catalyzed by the doxorubicin–iron complex. Biochemistry 21:1707–1713, 1982.
14. Bakowski M: ICRF 159, (+/-) 1,2-di(3,5-dioxopiperazin-1-yl)propane NSC 129943; razoxane. Cancer Treat Rev 3:95–107, 1976.
15. Repta A, Baltezor M, Bansal P: Utilization of an enantiomer as a solution to a pharmaceutical problem: Application to solubilization of 1,2-Di(4-piperazine-2,6-dione) propane. J Pharm Sci 65:238–242, 1976.
16. Dawson K: Studies on the cellular distribution of dioxopiperazines in cultured NHK-21S cells. Biochem Pharmacol 24:2249–2253, 1975.
17. Doroshow J, Burke T, Van Balgooy C, et al.: Cellular pharmacology of ICRF 187 in beating, doxorubicin-treated adult rat heart myocytes. Proc Am Assoc Cancer Res 31:442, 1990 (abstr).
18. Holcenberg J, Tutsch K, Earhart R, et al.: Phase I study of ICRF-187 in pediatric cancer patients and comparison of its pharmacokinetics in children and adults. Cancer Treat Rep 70:703–709, 1986.
19. Vats T, Kamen B, Krischer J: Phase II trial of ICRF-187 in children with solid tumors and acute leukemia. Invest New Drugs 9:333–337, 1991.
20. Hasinoff B: The interaction of the cardioprotective agent ICRF 187 ((+)-1,2-bis(3,5-dioxopiperazinyl-l-yl)propane); its hydrolysis product (ICRF 198); and other chelating agents with the Fe(III) and Cu(II) complexes of Adriamycin. Agents Actions 26:378–385, 1989.
21. Herman E, Ferrans V: Examination of the potential long-lasting protective effect of ICRF 187 against anthracycline-induced chronic cardiomyopathy. Cancer Treat Rev 17:155–160, 1990.
22. Herman E, Ardalan B, Bier C, et al.: Reduction of daunorubicin lethality and myocardial cellular alterations by pretreatment with ICRF 187 in Syrian golden hamsters. Cancer Treat Rep 63:89–92, 1979.
23. Herman E, Ferrans V, Young R, et al.: Effect of pretreatment with ICRF 187 on the total cumulative dose of doxorubicin tolerated by beagle dogs. Cancer Res 48:6918–6925, 1988.
24. Verhoef V, Colburn D, Bell V, et al.: Cardioprotective activity of ADR-529 for Daunorubicin and Idarubicin. Proc Am Assoc Cancer Res 31:404, 1990 (abstr).
25. Herman E, Ferrans V: ICRF 187 exerts cardioprotection when administered simultaneously with or 2 hours after doxorubicin in beagle dogs. Proc Am Assoc Cancer Res 31:404, 1990 (abstr).
26. Wadler S, Green M, Muggia F: Synergistic activity of doxorubicin and the bisdioxoperazine (+)-1,2-bis(3,5-dioxoperazinyl-l-yl)propane

(ICRF 187) against the murine sarcoma S180 cell line. Cancer Res 46:1176–1181, 1986.

27. Wadler S, Green M, Basch R, et al.: Lethal and sublethal effects of the combination of doxorubicin and the bisdiox-opiperazine, (+)-1,2-bis(3-5-dioxopoperazinyl-l-yl)propane (ICRF 187), on murine sarcoma S180 *in vitro*. Biochem Pharmacol 36:1495–1501, 1987.

28. Speyer J, Green M, Kramer E, et al.: Protective effect of the bispiperazinedione ICRF 187 against doxorubicin-induced cardiac toxicity in women with advanced breast cancer. N Engl J Med 319:745–752, 1988.

29. Speyer J, Green M, Zeleniuch-Jacquotte A, et al.: ICRF 187 permits longer treatment with doxorubicin in women with breast cancer. J Clin Oncol 10:117–127, 1992.

30. Steinherz L, Steinherz P, Tan C, Heller G, Murphy L: Cardiac toxicity 4 to 20 years after completing anthracycline therapy. J Am Med Assoc 266:1672–1677, 1991

31. Lipschultz S, Colan S, Walsh E, et al.: Ventricular tachycardia and sudden unexplained cardia death in late survivors of childhood malignancy treated with doxorubicin. Pediatr Res 27:145A, 1990 (abstr).

32. Lipschultz S, Conlan S, Sanders S, et al.: Late myocardial growth impairment in children treated with Adriamycin. Am J Cardiol 64:416, 1989 (abstr).

# 14. The Role of Genetic Counseling in the Management of Long-Term Survivors of Childhood Cancer

Judy E. Garber, M.D., M.P.H.

The existence of a genetic aspect to childhood cancers has long been recognized. Children with certain congenital anomalies and specific genetic syndromes have been shown to be at increased risk of developing particular cancers. Recent advances in molecular genetics have begun to expand the understanding of the genetic aspects of many disorders. The virtual explosion of genetic information and technologies will require that pediatric oncologists be increasingly cognizant of new issues facing patients and their families.

The success of treatment of childhood cancers has given pediatric oncologists the right to consider the complexities of the late effects of cancer treatment. Recognition of late toxicities may modify initial treatment strategies and influence recommendations for follow-up surveillance and counseling. Identification of individuals with significantly increased risks of developing late complications of cancer treatment could allow more precise individual tailoring of oncologic therapies and subsequent monitoring schemes.

There are multiple ways in which genetic information might influence the care of childhood cancer patients and their families. Among the questions raised by the availability of genetic diagnosis are:

1. Is a childhood cancer a manifestation of a genetic disorder that has other important nonneoplastic implications?

2. Does a genetic susceptibility to one cancer imply an increased risk of developing other neoplasms? Will radiation or chemotherapy influence that probability?

3. Do current cancer treatments create alterations in the genetic material in germ cells of patients that will be passed on and present as congenital anomalies, cancers, or other genetic disorders in the next generation?

4. What are the implications of genetic diagnosis for the family members of pediatric cancer patients? What about predictive testing?

5. What are the risks and benefits of opening Pandora's box? That is, what are some of the social and psychological issues that must be considered as the ability to obtain genetic information increases?

6. What other information is needed to make genetic counseling of patients and families most useful?

The discussion that follows attempts to address each of these questions and to provide examples of syndromes for which the answers are currently being sought.

The recognition of associations between clinically identifiable congenital and developmental anomalies and pediatric cancers antedate the molecular era in genet-

*Cardiac Toxicity After Treatment for Childhood Cancer*, pages 121–129, ©1993 Wiley-Liss, Inc.

ics. These observations contributed to the arrival of the modern era because of their value as markers of single-gene disorders. Children with tuberous sclerosis and Down's syndromes, the diagnoses of which are often apparent by physical examination early in life, are known to be at increased risk for the development of brain tumors and leukemia, respectively [1]. Alternatively, the diagnosis of Wilms' tumor might result in the recognition of a more subtle Beckwith-Wiedemann syndrome, or the diagnosis of a sarcoma in the identification of neurofibromatosis type I (NFI). The nononcologic implications of these disorders for the life of the child and his/her family are at least as important as the oncologic. Molecular diagnosis of NFI, for example, makes possible the recognition of less obvious forms of this highly variable syndrome, the clinical implications of which may differ from the more evident variants. Molecular techniques may thereby permit more precise definition of specific syndromes. They also may make possible prenatal diagnosis of a larger range of genetic disorders, though the clinical impact of these capacities is likely to be variable, depending on the extent to which a disorder has been recognized without them.

Recognition of an increased risk of cancer in association with an inherited syndrome is important for another reason. The goal of an improved ability to identify individuals at increased risk of cancer should be to improve cancer survival rates. Targeted surveillance with the hope of early intervention is likely an important strategy for achieving this goal. Direct benefits of medical testing of children for rare cancers may be difficult to demonstrate, as in the ultrasound surveillance of children with hemihypertrophy/Beckwith-Wiedemann syndrome for Wilms' tumor, but the paradigm remains.

An increased susceptibility to cancer may be the sole manifestation of a genetic alteration. Retinoblastoma is the prototype for this set of genetic disorders, many of which have been shown to involve tumor suppressor genes [2]. Genes in this class regulate cell cycling and suppress development of the neoplastic phenotype. Recognition of familial and nonfamilial forms of the disease led Knudson to the multihit model of cancer development, which predicted the existence of tumor suppressor genes [3]. In its simplest form, the model states that mutations in both alleles of a single genetic locus must be present to allow neoplastic transformation of a cell to occur. The first mutation can be either inherited (germline) or acquired (somatic); the second is virtually always acquired. Approximately 40% of children with retinoblastoma have the hereditary form of the disease (a germline alteration in one retinoblastoma gene). Early treatment of retinoblastoma is associated with excellent survival [4], but children with the inherited form of the disease are at greatly increased risk for the development of additional primary cancers. These include particularly bilateral retinoblastomas and osteosarcomas, but also soft tissue sarcomas, melanomas, and others, which are responsible for their excess mortality experience [5,6]. Moreover, the risk of multiple primary tumors increases substantially in the radiation therapy field [8] (Table 2).

Molecular genetic techniques will have great impact on the care of patients with hereditary retinoblastoma and their families. Bilateral cases are always heritable, but 10% to 12% of patients with unilateral retinoblastoma also will have a germline alteration. However, only 25% of children with hereditary retinoblastoma have a family history of the disease; the remaining 75% are the result of new mutations in germ cells [7]. Further, altered retinoblastoma genes may not be expressed as

**TABLE 1. Cancers in Single-Gene Syndromes With Noncancer Manifestations**

*Neurofibromatosis, type I*
Brain tumors
Sarcomas
Pheochromocytoma
*Beckwith-Wiedemann syndrome*
Wilms' tumor
Adrenocortical carcinoma
Hepatoblastoma
*Ataxia-telangiectasia*
Leukemia
*Familial adenomatous polyposis*
Colon carcinoma
Hepatoblastoma
Brain tumors (Turcot's)
Others

retinoblastoma tumors (incomplete penetrance); approximately 10% of obligate carriers of an altered gene will not develop the disease [7]. Specific molecular diagnosis is therefore extremely useful in distinguishing patients with the heritable form from among all patients with unilateral disease. It is also useful in identifying unaffected family members who have a germline alteration in their retinoblastoma gene [9].

The information gained is important to patients and family members in several ways. First, patients who are found to have the hereditary form of the disease are at dramatically increased risk of second primary malignancies, particularly after radiation therapy [6,8] (Table 2). To preserve vision, many will continue to be irradiated, using specialized techniques, until alternative treatments can be developed. These children must be followed indefinitely. Patients with sporadic disease have minimal risk of developing second cancers. These children and their siblings, as well as noncarrier siblings of patients with heritable disease, can also be spared intensive surveillance for the development of (additional) retinoblastomas. Surveillance entails examinations under anesthesia with attendant risks, expense, and anxiety [9].

Recognition of the role of radiation therapy in increasing the risk of second cancers in retinoblastoma survivors raises questions. There is likely an overrepresentation of patients with genetically determined cancer susceptibility among patients with multiple primary neoplasms. Patients with second primary cancers af-

**TABLE 2. Radiation, Chemotherapy, and Genetic Susceptibility Second Cancer Risk in All Pediatric Patients, All Except Genetic Retinoblastoma Patients and in Genetic Retinoblastoma Patients[a]**

| Patient Group | Radiation | ChemoRx | Tumors | 1RR |
|---|---|---|---|---|
| All | | | Any | 4.5 |
| All except genetic RB | - | - | Any | 3.9 |
| | + | - | Any | 5.6 |
| | + | + | Any | 9.3 |
| Genetic RB | - | | Any | 13.0 |
| | | | Bone | 174.0 |
| | + | - | Any | 26.0 |
| | | | Bone | 340.0 |
| | + | + | Any | 78.0 |
| | | | Bone | 771.0 |

[a]Data from Hawkins et al. [8].

ter childhood malignancy have shown a greater probability of carrying germline p53 alterations (see below) than other groups, though the series are highly selected [10,11]. Alkylating agent chemotherapy has also been associated with second tumor development [12]. Early identification of patients with a hereditary cancer predisposition may influence the development and application of alternative therapeutic strategies. These would be designed to limit exposure to carcinogenic treatment modalities, though compromise of therapeutic efficacy must remain a concern.

The known mutagenic properties of several classes of chemotherapeutic agents and radiation therapy has given rise to concern about their potential influence on the offspring of treated cancer survivors. These influences may become manifest as either excess cancer or congenital anomalies. Several studies have addressed these issues. In a large retrospective cohort study, Mulvihill and colleagues studied the offspring of 2,283 childhood cancer survivors and 3,604 sibling controls identified from five tumor registries [13]. No overall excess of cancer in the offspring of survivors was observed. Several cancers conformed with or resembled single-gene traits or recognized patterns of familial cancers (retinoblastoma, MEN2a). The cohort was also assessed for congenital anomalies as evidence of single-gene disorders that may have been related to treatment of the survivor; no excess was demonstrated [14]. Hawkins compared the birth outcomes of 2,286 childhood cancer survivors to population-based controls and could find no indication of germ cell mutation in the cases; other adverse outcomes were related to abdominal radiation [15]. Treatment with dactinomycin was implicated in cardiac malformations among survivor offspring in a study by Green et al. that failed to demonstrate an overall

effect of chemotherapy [16]. Others have not observed the dactinomycin effect [17]. Studies in this area may be limited by their relatively short follow-up and the small doses and limited number of chemotherapeutic agents to which the cohorts were exposed compared to current practice. They nonetheless provide some reassurance about the general resistance of the gonads to the potential mutagenic effects of antineoplastic treatment.

Consideration of treatment-associated risks and benefits for patients with enhanced cancer susceptibility involves decisions made between physician and patient family in the best interests of the patient. However, the possible existence of a heritable factor in the patient may often have implications for other family members as well.

Direct benefit to a relative may result from recognition of a previously undiagnosed syndrome in which early cancer diagnosis is beneficial. This is the case for multiple endocrine neoplasia, type 2A, a rare autosomal dominantly inherited syndrome of adult-onset medullary thyroid carcinoma (MTC) and pheochromocytoma [18].

Medullary thyroid cancer is often a highly lethal tumor, but its early identification and removal reduces the risk of subsequent metastatic disease [19]. The efficacy of screening family members for MTC with provocative pentagastrin stimulation of calcitonin secretion has led to its routine adoption in appropriate families [20,21]. However, the test must be repeated at regular intervals, and is potentially less informative for younger subjects. Issues of cost and compliance with screening add to the motives for better delineation of family members at genetic risk for the syndrome because they are at higher risk than those who merely have a family history of the disorder. A combination of genetic techniques (restriction fragment length polymorphism analysis) and provocative testing has been shown to provide the most accurate means of identifying at-risk individuals in appropriate families [21,22]. However, genetic testing is not always feasible. As the gene for MEN2a, mapped to chromosome 10 [23], has not yet been cloned, testing requires the cooperation of other family members. This can be a delicate and ethically complex requirement; some kindreds will be uninformative for other reasons.

Inherited cancer susceptibility syndromes in which childhood cancers are more prominent may have different implications for families already burdened by one child with cancer. Demonstration of a link between childhood sarcoma and maternal breast cancer has raised questions of timing and obligation [24]. When should a woman coping with sarcoma in her child be told of her increased breast cancer risk? What is the magnitude of the risk? Will early mammographic screening reduce breast cancer mortality in these mothers, or should prophylactic mastectomy be considered? A woman's reaction to news of her own increased cancer risk may well be influenced by her child's response to treatment, other experiences with cancer, and other life experience.

Some kindreds with childhood sarcoma and maternal breast cancer may be variants of the Li-Fraumeni syndrome. Here, an autosomal dominantly inherited cancer predisposition is manifest in the appearance of sarcomas, breast cancers, and other diverse cancers in childhood and young adulthood [25]. Germline alterations in the p53 tumor suppressor gene have been demonstrated in a proportion of these families [26,27]. Identification of a p53 mutation in a childhood cancer patient may have complex implications for close family members. When the alteration is the result of a new mutation in a germline p53 gene (not carried by either parent), there would be only the smallest chance for another child in the family to develop a childhood cancer as well, issues of nonpaternity aside. If the affected child survives his/her cancer, and there is no evidence to suggest a high cancer risk in offspring, then issues of reproduction will remain for him or her to decide. If, however, a parent were also found to carry the p53 alteration, then the probability of each child inheriting the same p53 alteration is 50%. Altered p53 gene carriers may have a 90% probability of developing cancer by age 60 years, with a 50% risk by age 30 years [28]. The diverse tumors for which carriers of the altered gene are at risk from birth are not limited to those for which useful surveillance measures are estab-

**TABLE 3. Some Familial Cancer Syndromes, Cancer Susceptibility Genes, Chromosomal Locations, and Associated Tumor Types[a]**

| Syndrome | Gene | Location | Tumors |
|---|---|---|---|
| Familial polyposis | APC | 5q | Hepatoblastoma, gastrointestinal, thyroid, ampullary |
| Neurofibromatosis I | NF1 | 17q | Nervous system sarcomas |
| Neurofibromatosis II | NF2 | 22q | Acoustic neuroma |
| Gorlin's syndrome | GS | 9q | Basal cell carcinoma, medulloblastoma |
| Li-Fraumeni syndrome | p53 | 17p | Sarcomas, leukemias, brain tumors, adrenal cortical, germ cell, breast, others |
| Multiple endocrine neoplasia 2a | MEN2a | 10 | Medullary thyroid, pheochromocytoma |

[a][23,41–44]

lished. The implicated malignant diseases include leukemias, brain tumors, and soft tissue and osteosarcomas [25,28].

It is now possible to determine the status of the p53 genes of cancer-free relatives of patients found to carry germline alterations in their p53 genes. This testing of unaffected persons for their status with respect to a particular gene is called *predictive testing*. It has been available for several years for disorders such as MEN2a, polycystic kidney disease, and Huntington's disease (HD). Predictive testing has only recently become available for syndromes of inherited cancer susceptibility. In predictive testing, an unaffected, disease-free individual seeks to learn his or her probability of carrying the altered form of a gene that in his or her family has been associated with a particular disease syndrome. Therefore, healthy members of Li-Fraumeni syndrome (LFS) families (which serves as the paradigm for other inherited cancer syndromes for the remainder of the discussion) can now find out whether they have an extraordinary risk of cancer or whether their risk is more like that of the general population.

This is clearly powerful information, and its potential impact should not be underestimated [29,30]. The possible benefits of determining an individual's status with respect to a cancer gene fall into two basic categories: reduction of anxiety and avoidance of cancer (Table 4). If uncertainty about one's cancer risk is disturbing, then relief of uncertainty may be a sufficient goal of testing. This is the case for HD, a degenerative neurologic disorder that is untreatable. For LFS, however, individuals shown to carry the altered gene associated with cancer risk can do something about it. They can be targeted for surveillance programs (like MEN2a), be counseled regarding avoidance of known or suspected carcinogens in occupational and recreational environments, and be edu-

**TABLE 4.  Predictive Testing: Potential Risks and Benefits**

*Risks*
Increased anxiety, depression, isolation, stigmatization
Alterations in family relationships
Problems with health and life insurability
Discrimination in educational and employment opportunities
*Benefits*
Relief from the anxiety of uncertainty
Opportunities for early diagnosis and improved surveillance to ultimately reduce cancer mortality
Preparedness to avoid recognized cancer risks
Prevention opportunities
Reproductive planning

cated regarding prevention strategies. These interventions are intended to facilitate early cancer diagnosis and cancer prevention, thereby reducing both cancer incidence and mortality for members of these families. Individuals shown not to carry the altered gene do not have the increased cancer risk. They thus would be able to avoid the psychological and financial burdens of intensive programs directed toward early detection, particularly of rare tumors. The genetic information would be useful for reproductive planning for either group in any case.

Basic ethical principles underlying genetic practice, autonomy and beneficence, must still apply, even if there were no potential risks to predictive testing. Not all patients will want to know about their genetic status, and the availability of the technology should not force them to learn it [31]. Moreover, there are surely potential adverse consequences to learning one's increased risk of developing cancer (Table 4). These have been carefully addressed in the HD predictive testing programs. For example, the anxiety associated with knowing that one has the predisposing gene may be greater than the anxiety of the unknown. Among HD carriers, however, increased depression without suicide in the early months after disclosure of positive test results has gradually diminished with time [32]. Unanticipated adverse experiences among noncarriers have been reported as well, and include "survivor guilt" [33]. Predictive testing programs for HD may have fared as well as they have because of decisions to include extensive psychological assessment before a blood specimen for testing is even taken. HD testing programs also provide access to further counseling following disclosure of test results [32–34]. The information from predictive testing is likely to influence already complex family relationships in unique ways, often raising challenging ethical concerns [35]. The burdens of the unrelated partners of family members with heritable conditions will also increase, and must be considered [36].

Perhaps more difficult to contain are the potential external ramifications of becoming aware of this aspect of one's genetic endowment. There is great concern over the absence of adequate protection of the privacy of genetic information. The federal government is beginning to design legislation to address this problem [37]. In the United States in 1992, persons shown to carry a cancer-predisposing gene may lose access to health and life insurance, and may suffer employment and opportunity discrimination [37,38]. Noncarriers may be freed of these same burdens by virtue of having eliminated a family cancer history from their risk consideration, if the information is correctly understood.

These issues become even more complex when predictive testing is extended to children. The HD programs have been restricted to adults, since the disease has onset only in adulthood, and the benefits of imparting early knowledge of carrier status to children can hardly be demonstrated [39]. Conversely, retinoblastoma programs have concentrated on children,

since the therapeutic benefits of early recognition of mutation carriers are nearly limited to very young children. The requirement for anticipated accrual of benefits of testing directly to the individuals to be tested comes again from the demand for autonomy in genetic practice [39]. Here, it is the children themselves who must gain; testing is not only for the relief of the anxiety of parents. There are nonetheless worrisome potential risks to children as well. They include all of the consequences that pertain to adults, along with fundamental alterations in family relationships, discrimination in educational opportunities, and stigmatization [30,39]. The affected child may be treated differently within the family, with potential loss of parent–child or sib–sib relationships, or there may be a limitation of resources extended to the child shown to be at increased risk [39]. These concerns have led some to suggest delaying testing until children are old enough to participate actively in the decision, and have an understanding of potential ramifications. A consensus conference concerning LFS recommended delaying testing of children until experience in adults can be evaluated [29,30]. However, in LFS, approximately 40% of cancers in reported families have occurred in persons aged 18 and younger [25]. It remains unknown as yet whether foreknowledge of p53 status will permit earlier detection and improved survival from the pediatric cancers seen in the syndrome. It is nonetheless difficult to contemplate withholding the potential benefits of early testing from children. All this makes it clear that even greater care is indicated when the inclusion of children is contemplated [30].

More precise information regarding the risks conferred by cancer-susceptibility genes would make counseling more useful. Identification of a p53 alteration, for example, does not predict where, when, what type, or even whether cancer will develop in a carrier. Investigation into the potential influences of environmental exposures or chemopreventive agents on cancer development in gene carriers is just beginning. The favorable or unfavorable experience of a survivor or that of a family with cancer is likely to influence decisions regarding predictive or prenatal testing at least as much as the information provided by professionals [40].

The identification of cancer-predisposing genes and the ability to perform predictive testing for their presence is new. It is expanding and may revolutionize cancer care in the future. Gene therapies will take these discoveries to their ultimate utility. Even before then, however, the ability to identify individuals at significantly increased risk of cancer on whom to focus surveillance and prevention energies will have an impact. It can be expected to exert an important influence on the care of cancer patients and their families. Childhood cancers are more likely to be manisfestations of cancer-susceptibility genes than are late-onset malignancies [3]. As a result, the interface between oncology and genetics may fall more often to the pediatric oncology team and confer an additional dimension to its roles in the care of childhood cancer patients and their families.

# REFERENCES

1. Miller RW: Genes, syndromes and cancer. Pediatr Rev 8:153–158, 1986.
2. Sager R: Tumor suppressor genes: The puzzle and the promise. Science 246:1406–1412, 1989.
3. Knudson AG Jr: Hereditary cancer, oncogenes, and anti-oncogenes. Cancer Res 45:1437–1443, 1985.
4. Abramson DH: Retinoblastoma 1990: Diagnosis, treatment and implications. Pediatr Ann 19:387–395, 1990.
5. Abramson DH, Ellsworth RM, Kitchin FD, Tung G: Second nonocular tumors in retinoblastoma survivors. Ophthalmology 91:1351–1355, 1984.
6. Eng C, Li FP, Abramson DH, et al.: Mortality from second tumors among long-term survivors of retinoblastoma. J Natl Cancer Inst (in press).
7. Vogel F: Genetics of retinoblastoma. Hum Genet 52:1–54, 1979.
8. Hawkins MM, Draper GJ, Kingston JE: Incidence of second primary tumours among childood cancer survivors. Br J Cancer 56:339–347, 1987.
9. Yandell DW, Campbell TA, Dayton SH, et al.: Oncogenic point mutations in the human retinoblastoma gene: Their application to genetic counseling. N Engl J Med 321:1689–1695, 1989.
10. Malkin D, Jolly KW, Barbier N, et al.: Germline mutations of the p53 tumor-suppressor gene in children and young adults with second malignant neoplasms. N Engl J Med 326:1309–1315, 1992.
11. Toguchida J, Yamaguchi T, Dayton SH, et al.: Prevalence and spectrum of germline mutations of the p53 gene among patients with sarcoma. N Engl J Med 326:1301–1308, 1992.
12. Tucker MA, D'Angio GJ, Boice JD Jr, et al.: Bone sarcomas linked to radiotherapy and chemotherapy in children. N Engl J Med 317:588–593, 1987.
13. Mulvihill JJ, Myers MH, Connelly RR, et al.: Cancer in offspring of long-term survivors of childhood and adolescent cancer. Lancet 814–817, 1987.
14. Mulvihill JJ, Byrne J, Steinhorn SA, et al.: Genetic disease in offspring of cancer in the young. Am J Hum Genet 39(Suppl):A72, 1986.
15. Hawkins MM: Is there evidence of a therapy-related increase in germ cell mutation among childhood cancer survivors? J Nat Cancer Inst 83:1643–1650, 1991.
16. Green DM, Zevon MA, Lowrie G, et al.: Congenital anomalies in children of patients who received chemotherapy for cancer in childhood and adolescence. N Engl J Med 325:141–146, 1991.
17. Byrne J, Nicholson HS, Mulvihill JJ: Absence of birth defects in offspring of women treated with dactinomycin. N Engl J Med 326:137, 1992.
18. Schimke RN: Genetic aspects of multiple endocrine neoplasia. Annu Rev Med 35:25–31, 1984.
19. Gagel RF, Tashjian AH Jr, Cummings T, et al.: The clinical outcome of prospective screening for multiple endocrine neoplasia type 2a. N Engl J Med 318:478–484, 1988.
20. Melvin KEW, Miller HH, Tashijian AH Jr: Early diagnosis of medullary carcinoma of the thyroid gland by means of calcitonin assay. N Engl J Med 285:1115–1120, 1971.
21. Ponder BAJ, Coffey R, Gagel RF, et al.: Risk

estimates and screening in families of patients with medullary thyroid carcinoma. Lancet 397–401, 1988.

22. Sobol H, Narod SA, Nakamura Y, et al.: Screening for multiple endocrine neoplasia type 2a with DNA-polymorphism analysis. N Engl J Med 321:996–1001, 1989.

23. Simpson NE, Kidd KK, Goodfellow PJ, et al.: Assignment of multiple endocrine neoplasia type 2a to chromosome 10 by linkage. Nature 328:528–530, 1987.

24. Birch JM, Hartley AM, Marsden HB, et al.: Excess risk of breast cancer in the mothers of children with soft tissue sarcomas. Br J Cancer 49:325–331, 1984.

25. Li FP, Fraumeni JF Jr, Mulvihill JJ, et al.: A cancer family syndrome in twenty-four kindreds. Cancer Res 48:5358–5362, 1988.

26. Malkin D, Li FP, Strong LC, et al.: Germ line p53 mutations in a familial syndrome of breast cancer, sarcomas, and other neoplasms. Science 250:1233–1238, 1990.

27. Srivastava S, Zou Z, Pirollo K, et al.: Germline transmission of a mutated p53 gene in a cancer-prone family with Li-Fraumeni syndrome. Nature 348:747–749, 1990.

28. Strong LC, Williams WR, Tainsky MA: The Li-Fraumeni syndrome: From clinical epidemiology to molecular genetics. Am J Epidemiol 135:190–199, 1992.

29. Li FP, Correa P, Fraumeni JF Jr: Testing for germ line p53 mutations in cancer families. Cancer Epidemiol Biomark Prev 1:91–94, 1991.

30. Li FP, Garber JE, Friend SH, et al.: Recommendations on predictive testing for germ line p53 mutations among cancer-prone individuals. J Nat Cancer Inst 84:1156–1160, 1992.

31. Clarke A: Is non-directive genetic counseling possible? Lancet 338:998–1001, 1991.

32. Bloch M, Adam S, Wiggins S, Huggins M, Hayden MR: Predictive testing for Huntington disease in Canada: The experience of those receiving an increased risk. Am J Med Genet 42:499–507, 1992.

33. Huggins M, Bloch M, Wiggins S, et al.: Predictive testing for Huntington disease in Canada:

Adverse effects and unexpected results in those receiving a decreased risk. Am J Med Genet 42:508–515, 1992.

34. Brandt J, Quaid KA, Folstein SE, et al.: Presymptomatic diagnosis of delayed-onset disease with lined DNA markers. The experience with Huntington disease. J Am Med Assoc 261:3108–3114, 1989.

35. Huggins M, Bloch M, Kanani SH, et al.: Ethical and legal dilemmas arising during predictive testing for adult-onset disease: The experience of Huntington disease. Am J Hum Genet 47:4–12, 1990.

36. Tibben A, Vegter-VD, Vlis M, et al.: Testing for Huntington disease with support for all parties. Lancet 335:553, 1990.

37. Billings PR, Kohn MA, de Cueva M, et al.: Discrimination as a consequence of genetic testing. Am J Hum Genet 50:476–482, 1992.

38. Council on Ethical and Judicial Affairs, American Medical Association. Use of genetic testing by employers. J Am Med Assoc 266:1827–1830, 1991.

39. Bloch M, Hayden MR: Opinion: Predictive testing for Huntington disease in childhood: Challenges and implications. Am J Hum Genet 46:1–4, 1990.

40. Leonard CO, Chase GA, Childs B: Genetic counseling: A consumers' view. N Engl J Med 287:433–439, 1972.

41. Nishisho I, Nakamura Y, Miyoshi Y, et al.: Mutations of chromosome 5q21 genes in FAP and colorectal cancer patients. Science 253:665–669, 1991.

42. Barker D, Wright E, Nguyen K, et al.: Gene for von Recklinghausen neurofibromatosis is in the pericentromeric region of chromosome 17. Science 236:1100–1102, 1987.

43. Wertelecki W, Rouleau GA, Superneau DW, et al.: Neurofibromatosis 2: Clinical and DNA linkage studies of a large kindred. N Engl J Med 319:278–283, 1988.

44. Gailani MR, Bale SJ, Leffell DJ, et al.: Developmental defects in Gorlin syndrome related to a putative tumor suppressor gene on chromosome 9. Cell 69:111–117, 1992.

# Index